RAPID WEIGHT I

FOR WOMEN

Lose weight fast with healthy and powerful mini habits. Stop emotional eating and increase your self-confidence with guided meditations and positive affirmations

SELF HELP HABITS

Copyright 2020 - All rights reserved.

The content contained within this book may not be reproduced, duplicated or transmitted without direct written permission from the author or the publisher.

Under no circumstances will any blame or legal responsibility be held against the publisher, or author, for any damages, reparation, or monetary loss due to the information contained within this book. Either directly or indirectly.

Legal Notice:

This book is copyright protected. This book is only for personal use. You cannot amend, distribute, sell, use, quote or paraphrase any part, or the content within this book, without the consent of the author or publisher.

Disclaimer Notice:

Please note the information contained within this document is for educational and entertainment purposes only. All effort has been executed to present accurate, up to date, and reliable, complete information. No warranties of any kind are declared or implied. Readers acknowledge that the author is not engaging in the rendering of legal, financial, medical or professional advice. The content within this book has been derived from various sources. Please consult a licensed professional before attempting any techniques outlined in this book. By reading this document, the reader agrees that under no circumstances is the author responsible for any losses, direct or indirect, which are incurred as a result of the use of information contained within this document, including, but not limited to, — errors, omissions or inaccuracies.

Table of content

INTRODUCTION 6

CHAPTER 1: WHAT IS HYPNOSIS 9

What is Hypnosis? 10
How Does Hypnosis Work? 13
Common Misconceptions About Hypnosis 15
What Can Be Achieved with Hypnosis 17
The Betty Erickson Method 17
Benson method 21

CHAPTER 2: WHAT IS HYPNOSIS FOR WEIGHT LOSS? 25

How does Food Invade our Minds? 26
How Hypnotherapy Helps you Lose Weight 29

CHAPTER 3: IS MEDITATION THE SAME AS SELF HYPNOSIS? 32

What is Meditation? 32
What is Self-Hypnosis? 34
Similarities Between Meditation and Self-Hypnosis 35
The Difference Between Meditation and Self-Hypnosis 35

CHAPTER 4: SLEEP DEPRIVATION AND WEIGHT GAIN 40

BETTER HABITS TO IMPROVE YOUR SLEEP 43

CHAPTER 5: EMOTIONAL EATING AND OVEREATING 48

THE PSYCHOLOGY OF EMOTIONAL EATING 49
COMMON CAUSES OF EMOTIONAL EATING 50

CHAPTER 6: WEIGHT LOSS HYPNOSIS 56

CHAPTER 7: HOW TO PREPARE YOURSELF FOR HYPNOSIS 60

CHAPTER8: WEIGHT LOSS HYPNOSIS SESSION 63

SELF-HYPNOSIS FOR WEIGHT LOSS SCRIPT 1 63
SELF-HYPNOSIS FOR WEIGHT LOSS SCRIPT 2 69
SELF-HYPNOSIS FOR WEIGHT LOSS SCRIPT 3 74
MEDITATION FOR WEIGHT LOSS 77

CHAPTER 9: DEEP SLEEP HYPNOSIS 80

WHAT IS DEEP SLEEP HYPNOSIS? 80
DEEP SLEEP FOR WEIGHT LOSS 81

CHAPTER 10: HOW TO PREPARE YOURSELF TO SLEEP HYPNOSIS 85

WHAT TO DO BEFORE BEDTIME 86
THE ENVIRONMENT 88

THE RIGHT POSTURE 89

CHAPTER 11: MEDITATION TO CALM AN OVERACTIVE MIND 92

CHAPTER 12: MEDITATIONS FOR RELAXATION AND SELF-IMAGE 96

CHAPTER 13: DEEP SLEEP HYPNOSIS 109

CHAPTER 14: MEDITATION FOR DEEPER AND HEALTHIER SLEEP 122

MEDITATION FOR A FULL NIGHT'S SLEEP 122

CHAPTER 15: DEEP SLEEP HYPNOSIS 2 128

CHAPTER 16: OVERCOME MENTAL BLOCKS TO LOSE WEIGHT 137

METABOLISM 137
HOW TO OVERCOME MENTAL BLOCKS 140
WHY PRACTICE MEDITATION AND AFFIRMATIONS? 141
HOW DO YOU USE POSITIVE AFFIRMATIONS IN MEDITATION? 143

CHAPTER 17: GUIDED MEDITATIONS 146

MEDITATION FOR HEALTHIER HABITS 146
MEDITATION FOR POSITIVE THINKING 148
MEDITATION TO COPE DURING DIFFICULT TIMES 154

CHAPTER 18: LOVE YOUR BODY, LOVE YOUR SOUL 163

IS YOUR WEIGHT YOUR BAROMETER FOR HAPPINESS? 165

POSITIVE AFFIRMATIONS FOR WEIGHT LOSS 167

AFFIRMATIONS FOR SELF-LOVE 170

AFFIRMATIONS FOR SELF-ESTEEM 172

SIMPLE DAILY GOOD HABITS 174

CONCLUSION 185

Introduction

In a supersized world, people have too many options to eat and drink, but what is behind overweight is often more than the desire for a wide variety of potato chips. The diet has developed around obesity, forcing overweight people to pay a high price for expensive and risky diets, pills, or operations, by cutting out carbs or fats, taking pills or injections, performing surgeries, or drinking miracle potions. A lot of dieters lose weight temporarily, but don't change the mindset that contributes to weight gain. The result is that after all the hard work and potentially spending thousands of dollars, most dieters regain their weight and feel even more frustrated.

The healthiest and most effective way to lose weight is not the fastest. For those who want to maintain a healthy weight and healthily lose body fat, weight loss hypnosis is what you should consider.

Weight loss should be smooth without constant hunger and constant cravings for food. Weight loss hypnosis is an effective way to lose weight because it is easy to retrain your subconscious, and you can see the results immediately. Weight loss hypnosis can help you change your emotions and control your poor diet.

Hypnosis has helped people lose weight sustainably by changing the way they think about their eating habits, reducing stress and pressure, and learning to relax. Overeating has nothing to do with hunger, but rather a high level of stress and other negative emotional feelings that allow food to distract from that feeling.

Like all hypnosis, weight loss hypnosis proposes weight loss while people are in a relaxed state, as long as the suggestions correspond first of all to what the person wants to do. Part of the focus is on changing preferences and choices for a better alimentation, and to overcome appetite.

Since many dieters have negative thinking patterns that encourage them to use junk food to change their feelings, hypnosis for weight loss also helps you to see yourself as a healthy person that does not need food to change anything. You learn to see changes in eating habits not as a hardship, but as empowerment because that is what you want to do in the first place.

Chapter 1:
What is Hypnosis

The subconscious is the part of the mind with which we want to communicate under hypnosis. This is your true self, your real personality. It is literal and works in schemas or programs. It is thousands of percent more powerful than your conscious mind. You can think of your subconscious in several ways.

It is a powerful computer that runs on programming and that programming could be good, bad, or "I'll kill you" programming. It doesn't rationalize anything. (Remember work is done in the conscious mind) If there is a program in your subconscious that says something like "Food equals Comfort," you will have a hard time losing weight unless you find and disable that program! Side note here, for many people, food offers the same comfort and safety. If babies are scared, tired, irritable, or just bother us, we put something in their mouths (food or a pacifier). Thus, the program, Food = Comfort, was born and strengthened.

Permanent memory. An exciting part of the subconscious mind is the fact that this is where its permanent memory resides. It memorized every moment, every event in your life, and this goes back to five months ago, in the womb before birth! It has archived everything you have seen, touched, smelled, heard, and experienced in your entire life.

Finding and removing a deep-seated problem comes down to circumventing that critical factor. You can think of this critical factor as if it were a watchdog.

When you are awake, he is awake and on guard. He says, "Wow, I like what I'm hearing, but it doesn't correspond to current programming, so I'll reject it." This means that the person likes what they hear and can be useful for a short time, but in the end, it will not change it.

Herein lies the power of hypnosis! You can think of hypnosis as letting the watchdog sleep for a while and then whispering new positive suggestions for a change in his ear. When the hypnosis session ends, "Because of three, the eye wide open and fully alert, one, two, three" - that watchdog returns, instead, but something has changed. The new program is now online! You have put a perception of the critical factor in everything in your world.

In short, the unconscious mind is powerful and automatic. It is responsible for almost everything we do every day, for better or for worse. For centuries, hypnosis has provided us with a way to access our unconscious thoughts and provide more accurate and positive information to use.

What is Hypnosis?

Now that we understand how our mind works, let's start talking about hypnosis. Hypnosis is a relaxation technique, in which we follow the steps to achieve a state of higher concentration and relaxation. This is called a "hypnotic state" and is similar to daydreaming or the feeling of losing track of time after driving for long periods of time (called "road hypnosis").

Under hypnosis, we are still very much and in control. In the hypnotic state, you are only relaxed and highly focused. This allows you to achieve a high state of consciousness. In the hypnotic state, the mind is highly suggestible. That's why hypnosis is so powerful.

Most bad habits, negative inclinations, and phobias are all triggered by our unconscious thoughts. A smoker tends to have automatic cravings, which triggers the conscious mind to reach for a cigarette. But under hypnosis, the smoker can reformulate these unconscious impulses. First, he/she must figure out the triggers of these automatic thoughts to begin with. And then, start removing and replacing them with more positive associations.

In other words, positive thoughts are pushed to the front of the unconscious and stifle the old way of thinking. This is why hypnosis works. It gets you to the root cause of your habit or fixation. Well, this is a very broad overview of what hypnosis is.

You probably have some unanswered questions. I will help you investigate hypnosis on a deeper level, including providing information on what hypnosis is, what actually happens in the brain during hypnosis, and what you can do to get started.

Understand What Hypnosis Is

Hypnosis is sometimes referred to as the hypnotic state. This is the relaxed and highly focused mental structure that you achieve after being hypnotized.

You can come to think of hypnosis as meditation with a goal. Both are similar in the sense that they will try to achieve a state of relaxation and concentration. But with hypnosis, you go one step further. In this state of intense awareness, you begin to examine your subconscious and receive suggestions that can help you reformulate and improve the functioning of the subconscious. The process generally includes three steps:

Phase #1: Hypnotic induction

The hypnotic induction is the first phase you must follow to achieve hypnosis. Usually, you will be sitting in a chair, lying on a bed, or anywhere comfortable with your eyes closed. You can also use a script and/or controlled breathing techniques to relax your mind and focus.

Phase #2: Hypnotic state

Now the hypnotic state is reached. In the hypnotic state, you feel physically and mentally relaxed; you are so calm and focused on heightened awareness.

Phase #3: Hypnotic suggestions

Once in hypnosis, your mind becomes highly suggestible. In this phase, your mind receives hypnotic suggestions. These suggestions are meant to replace and update old ways in your subconscious thoughts.

How Does Hypnosis Work?

I just showed you a breakdown of the phases of hypnosis. But how does hypnosis work? In hypnosis, we can reformulate our unconscious thoughts. You may wonder: why is the hypnotized mind so suggestible? What happens in the brain when we are hypnotized? Can everyone be hypnotized? The short answer is: we can likely all be hypnotized!

According to research, the majority of people, about 75-85 percent, can achieve a slight trance. And most of these people share some common traits such as:

- Daydream often
- Get absorbed in daily activities quickly.
- Show more empathy
- Are open-minded about hypnosis.

Of course, it is not necessary to show all or one of these to be hypnotized. But they offer more susceptibility to hypnosis. However, even for those who do not achieve a mild hypnotic state, there are still benefits to hypnosis. Hypnosis is a powerful tool for relaxing or improving the mind's susceptibility to positive reinforcement.

What happens to the brain?

Once we have bypassed the conscious mind, we can communicate directly with the subconscious. In other words, hypnosis allows you to go "under the hood" and access your subconscious mind. There are a lot of theories as to why hypnosis work. However, the relevant thought here is that hypnosis helps us achieve a state of deep concentration and relaxation, which allows us to avoid the conscious mind.

Recent research confirms part of this theory. One study showed that the areas of the brain responsible for critical thinking show reduced activity under hypnosis. Other studies on brain activity during hypnosis confirms that hypnosis allowed us to:

- Stimulates stimuli: This describes a reduced activity in the anterior dorsal cingulate of the brain. This part forms our awareness network. That is, under hypnosis, we can adjust our worries and stress. And we get absorbed in the experience.

- Increased mind-brain connections: studies show that the mind is more in tune with how it controls the body. This explains how hypnotic suggestions help us manage how our body responds to specific situations, such as overcoming fears, cravings, or negative responses.

- Reduced self-consciousness: Studies show the connection between two brain networks. This explains why we become much less aware of our actions, and therefore more suggestible.

Overall, this shows that our brains behave differently in the hypnotic state. In fact, many of these processes are unique to hypnosis.

What Does the hypnotic state feel like?

You may be wondering, "what exactly do I feel in the hypnotic state?" You could describe your feelings as being in deep relaxation or the trance state. You will feel hyper receptive but relaxed, as you would feel during meditation.

When entering hypnosis, you may feel some physical sensations such as relaxation and heaviness around your muscles, such as the eyelids. You can feel your body. You will bypass your conscious mind, enter your subconscious mind, and push out negative associations. Most people describe the hypnotic state as a feeling of having a nap. However, the difference is during hypnosis, you are conscious and guided through an experience.

Common Misconceptions About Hypnosis

Hypnosis is not a form of mind control. Instead, it is similar to meditation. Follow the steps that allow you to enter a state of deep concentration and relaxation. And you keep control of everything.

Unfortunately, pop culture has blurred the image of hypnosis and has led to some misconceptions. Common ones include:

Myth #1. You lose control

Hypnotized people are fully aware of their surroundings. And experience a high level of focus. They discard distractions, achieve relaxation, and finally calm the mind. There is no loss of control.

Myth #2. You are asleep or unconscious

The deep attention and relaxation achieved during hypnosis are often confused with sleep or unconsciousness. That is why the origin of the word hypnosis is the ancient Greek word "Hypnos," or sleep. But unlike sleep, you are conscious, in fact, extremely conscious.

Myth #3. You can get caught up in hypnosis

You saw it in the movies: someone experiences hypnosis for the first time and never wakes up. They remain hypnotized forever. This is pure fiction. You are in TOTAL control and can open your eyes and go back to the surroundings.

Myth #4. Hypnosis is a magic bullet

Hypnosis is not a cure. You have to make a difference and keep working on it. But if you want to improve, the researcher has shown that hypnosis can help.

What Can Be Achieved with Hypnosis

Your subconscious mind controls almost all of your thinking. About 95 percent of your thoughts are independently generated through the unconscious mind. This is why we get caught doing unwanted behaviors. They are deeply embedded in our minds due to repetition and reinforcement. Many of our fears, worries, habits, impulses, and doubts, therefore, remain unconscious.

Under hypnosis, we try to reformulate and reverse these "thought patterns. Therefore, hypnotherapy has been shown to be very useful for unconsciously motivating habits.

The Betty Erickson Method

Betty Erickson developed this hypnosis technique. Although Betty wasn't a hypnotist, she understood how our visual-auditory-kinesthetic systems influenced our world in a trance state. This technique has become increasingly popular in the world of hypnosis. This hypnosis technique can be used to relieve stress or any other self-hypnosis you would like to do.

The basic principles:

They are all thoughts in the form of images, full of sounds and emotions.

When we visualize, we think of all possible scenarios. We imagine how it is now, how we want it to be, and what it will be like in the future. This is simply a mixture of images that are already stored in the brain.

In the same way, our thoughts are associated with sounds, which are also the result of information stored in our minds, such as songs and sounds we imagine, speak, or hear. These sounds also include background noises and sounds we make when in dialogue with ourselves and others.

Emotions are the third way we think. These could be what we've experienced before or what we want to try or experience. Although our conscious mind uses these three, more often, only one is dominant. Therefore, for someone who associates his thoughts with sounds, he will not be as successful if he mainly uses visuals.

Before you move on to self-hypnosis, you may want to set goals for what you want to happen. Once you're ready, follow these steps.

Step 1: Get comfortable.

Sit or lie down in a quiet and comfortable position.

Relax your mind and body and feel yourself begin to wander in a state of relaxation. Let yourself in for a bit while staying on top of the outside world and keeping your eyes open, but you start to sleep.

Step 2: focus on something you are seeing.

Shadows moving across the wall or unique surroundings motifs can provide something unique to see. Be aware of what you see and become aware of it. Do it three different times, with three different objects.

Step 3: focus on something you are listening to

This could be the sound of your breathing, the wind brushing against the windows, or the hum of the air conditioner. Find three different things and observe them and bring them to your knowledge.

Step 4: focus on something you feel.

Maybe it's the movement of muscles along the joints, the gap between the shoulder blades, the weight of the feet on the floor, or the weight of the body on the chair. Consider three things and become aware of them.

Step 5: Continue with two things, then one thing.

Repeat steps 2-4, and this time, you will see two things, hear two things and feel two things. So, do the same for one thing.

Step 6: Close your eyes and go inward.

Allow yourself to go inward and relax and feel slightly drifting. This is a calm and peaceful state where you can simply let it go.

Step 7: imagine a new or old show

This could be what you saw before, or it could be something completely new. Imagine something you can see. Maybe it's a purple elephant, maybe it's a soothing blue light, or perhaps it's the sight of a ship taking off.

Step 8: imagine an old or new sound

You can create a sound, or it can be something you are already familiar with. An example is that you can hear the sound of an animal in nature, or a spacecraft suspended in space or the relaxing rain that falls on a group of leaves.

Step 9: imagine an old or new feeling

Become aware of something you've noticed before, or perhaps something you want to pay more attention to, such as how your breathing feels when it enters your lungs and the relaxation around your clavicle when you exhale.

Step 10: now, you are in hypnosis!

In this hypnotic state, you can make suggestions or just relax and let the ideas take effect that you had in mind before starting the session. The only trust that your mind is letting suggestions circulate: the more you can get carried away, the easier your ideas will take root inside.

Step 11: emerge

Say to yourself, "As I count from 1 to 5, I shall emerge with a great sense of energy, feeling refreshed and relaxed."

So, count from 1 to 5, allowing as much time as your body needs to make it real for you.

Benson method

The term "Relaxation Response" was developed by Dr. Herbert Benson. This response is defined as the ability to encourage your body to release chemicals and brain signals that slow down muscles and organs and increase blood flow to the brain.

Benson can be widely credited for demystifying meditation and helping to bring it into the mainstream by changing the name of meditation to "Response to Relaxation." His studies have been able to show that meditation promotes better health. People who meditate regularly experience lower stress levels, greater well-being, and can even lower blood pressure levels and resting heart rate.

In his book, The Response to Relaxation, Dr. Benson describes the scientific benefits of relaxation, explaining that regular relaxation response practice can be an effective treatment for a wide range of stress-related ailments.

The relaxation response is the opposite reaction to the "fight" response. The relaxation response practice is beneficial as it neutralizes the physiological effects of stress and the fight-or-flight response.

It is normal for people experiencing the fight/flight response to describe uncomfortable physiological changes, such as muscle tension, headache, stomach pain, rapid heartbeat, and shallow breathing.

The relaxation response is an effective way to deactivate the fight/flight response and return the body to pre-stress levels. Relaxation Response is a physical state of deep relaxation that involves the other part of our nervous system: the parasympathetic nervous system.

There are multiple ways to elicit the relaxation response. Pure relaxation can be achieved by moving away from daily thinking and choosing a word, sound, phrase, sentence, or concentrating on your breathing and focusing on it.

The best time for relaxation response practice is first thing in the morning for 10 to 20 minutes. Practicing just once or twice a day may be enough to counteract the stress response and bring deep relaxation and inner peace.

Steps for an explicit relaxation response

Sit quietly in a comfortable position.

Close your eyes

Deeply relaxes all muscles, from feet to face. Keep them relaxed. [Relax your tongue, and your thoughts will stop.]

Breathe through your nose. Become aware of your breathing. Breathe out, say the word "one" calmly to yourself. For instance, inhale, then exhale and say "one," enter and exit and repeat "one." Breathe easily and naturally.

Continue for 10-20 minutes. You can open your eyes to see the time, but you cannot use an alarm clock. When you are finished, sit quietly for a few minutes, initially with your eyes closed and then with your eyes open. Don't get up for a few minutes.

Don't worry if you can't achieve a deep level of relaxation. Maintain a passive attitude and allow relaxation at your own pace. When distracting thoughts creep in, try to ignore them by not dwelling on them and repeat "one" again.

With practice, the answer should come with little effort. Practice the technique once or twice a day, but not within two hours after each meal, as the body digestive processes seem to interfere with the activation of the Relaxation Response

Chapter 2: What is Hypnosis for Weight Loss?

Close your eyes, relax, with every breath you take, imagine inresistible cravings disappear, and your urge to overeat fading away. Visualize yourself no longer having the urge to console yourself with unhealthy snacks. You might begin to think, "if only weight loss this simple, and I could turn off my cravings!"

Well, that is the idea of hypnosis to lose weight. Under hypnosis, those seeking to lose weight have the power to update automatic thoughts that trigger the desire to eat. Overeating tends to be associated with certain feelings, relationships, and events in our minds. Our minds have convinced us that, in certain situations, food has an essential purpose, that is, to use it to relieve stress.

To achieve long-term weight loss, we must remove these unconscious barriers and replace these automatic thoughts with more useful information. Hypnosis allows us to access these automatic thoughts, eliminate negative associations, and develop positive associations that can help us achieve long-term success in weight loss.

How does Food Invade our Minds?

The food we eat has an unconscious and automatic response to stress. These kinds of mental habits are the main reasons why losing weight is a challenge for most of us. Let me explain…

Now, imagine starting a fad diet of which you are two weeks into already, and you're beginning to see some reasonable amount of weight loss and feel happy. But then something else changes. You got a new job, a new routine and now it's even more difficult for you to lose weight. You've less time to cook, you've stopped counting calories, and eat more unhealthy foods. Now, it's only a matter of time before you see yourself gaining weight and completely falling out of the diet.

What do you think went wrong? When we take a more in-depth look at it, we might discover a "habit pattern" that explains it. Habit patterns are formed through repetition over time, thereby becoming an automatic response to stimuli or the environment. And in this case, you probably developed an emotional eating habit that kept you from achieving your weight loss goals.

Deep in our unconscious minds, we develop a strong belief about unhealthy these unhealthy habits. Over time, we train our minds to believe that these habits are essential to maintain our well-being, making it challenging to achieve long-term weight loss success.

Most of these associations have a negative impact on our relationship with food. Some of which include:

- Using food as a source of comfort in times of stress or sadness.

- Eating to distract ourselves from feelings of anxiety, sadness, or anger.

- Overeating unhealthy and sugary food is associated with good times.

- Sugary and unhealthy foods as a reward for good deeds.

Achieving long-term weight loss success requires re-evaluating and understanding the root causes. And that is exactly where hypnosis comes into play.

Identifying why you are not achieving your weight loss goals is the first step you must take when using hypnosis to lose weight. And then, you through a process called 'induction" where your mind and body relax and enter into the state of hypnosis. Under hypnosis, your mind is highly suggestible. At this point, you've bypassed the conscious mind and can now speak directly to your unconscious mind.

In self-hypnosis, you will have suggestions, positive affirmations, while you visualize the changes. You can try it with weight loss hypnosis recordings! Here are some tips for weight loss hypnosis:

- Visualization of your success. Visualizing your success is very important if you must achieve your weight loss goals. Visualizing your success makes you know how it feels and will keep you going.

- Enhance confidence. Use positive affirmations to boost your confidence.

- Rename your inner voice. Under hypnosis, you're able to tame your inner voice that refuses to give up unhealthy food and make it an ally on your weight loss journey with positive affirmations.

- Touching the unconscious. Under hypnosis, you can be more aware of why you are making unhealthy food choices and lack portion control. This helps you establish a more conscious approach towards making good food choices.

- Avoid fear. Fear is one of the reasons why people never try in the first place. Under hypnosis, you can tame the fear of not succeeding and keep working on achieving your weight loss goals.

- Identification and requalification of habit patterns. Once in hypnosis, you can explore your relationship with food and disable those automatic responses. By constant repetition of positive affirmations, you can eliminate automatic and unhealthy habits.

- Develop a coping mechanism. Through hypnosis, you can re-establish healthier ways to handle stress and emotions.

- Try eating healthily. You can hypnotize yourself into being more comfortable with eating at home instead of a restaurant. This will make it easier for you to make healthier food choices.

- Making healthier food choices. We all want and love some unhealthy food. Under hypnosis, we can convince our minds to develop a preference for healthier food options. Which also has an impact on the portion size you choose.

- Increasing unconscious indicators. Through constant repetition, over and over again, we learn to block out the signals our body sends when it's full. Under hypnosis, we learn to become more aware of these indicators.

Your self-hypnosis plan should include suggestions that are more relevant to your relationship with food. This way, you could train your unconscious to slow down its automatic responses, while providing the unconscious with new and more useful ways to handle stress and emotions.

How Hypnotherapy Helps you Lose Weight

Under hypnosis, our minds are much more open to suggestions. Studies have proven some interesting changes in the brain during hypnosis, which allow us to learn without consciously thinking about the information we are receiving. In other words, we are bypassing the conscious mind!

When the conscious mind receives hypnotic suggestions, it doesn't question what it is hearing. And this is how hypnosis helps to break through these barriers that have kept us from losing weight.

I must emphasize that the barriers in our minds are strong, and only through repeated work we can successfully breakthrough and reformulate these beliefs. However, repeated hearing positive statements and suggestions about healthy eating are the first steps on your journey to weight loss. You are training your mind to think differently

Chapter 3:
Is Meditation the Same as Self Hypnosis?

Many people confuse one of these terms with the other, and authors tend to make this problem worse by using them interchangeably in their writing. Meditation and Self-hypnosis are relaxing and a very effective way to reduce stress and calm the mind and body. However, there are crucial differences. Let's take a closer look at these two related but different relaxation methods.

What is Meditation?

Meditation is a relaxation technique to calm the mind. It can be achieved by focusing on something specific. It can be your breath, an object, or a particular phrase or word. When you meditate with your eyes open, you generally focus on an object in the room. On the other hand, if you meditate with your eyes closed, you more likely to focus on your breathing or repeat a specific phrase or word. This is called "mantra," and it is usually repeated either silently or out loud.

Focusing on something specific is an essential feature of meditation; therefore, when thoughts arise, you will notice them briefly. Once you do, you want to quickly and carefully return your attention to the center of your meditation practice.

The Aim of Meditation

The main goal of meditation is to calm your mind and make you feel calmer. This will help you feel happier and relax. It helps you to be more present, and it's also great to improve concentration by focusing on one thing. You will notice more of your thoughts and feelings with improved self-awareness.

Meditation helps you reach a calm state of mind or perhaps an altered state of consciousness. It happens when beta brain waves (our normal active brain state) go to the alpha level: meditation is often part of a broader spiritual practice.

Meditation may or may not be guided. Guided meditation requires listening to a recording (or a person). Become your center of focus. The voice then guides you to focus on different things. It can be your breath, different parts of your body, or positive words and phrases. You can also add guided imagery to help you relax with your imagination.

With unguided meditation, you do it yourself, focusing on your breathing, an object, or a mantra. Meditation is incredibly easy to learn and do. You focus on one thing and notice what your mind is doing. And you can meditate almost anywhere!

In my opinion, guided meditations are very similar to self-hypnosis recordings. Either way, focus your mind on the content of the record.

With guided meditations, the purpose of the suggestions is to help you achieve a calmer mind. A self-hypnosis recording can also do this, but it will often focus on changing a habit, behavior, or experience of something you want to happen in your imagination.

Guided meditation can also help you reprogram your subconscious as well as self-hypnosis recording. Both reach the relaxed state necessary to take into account positive ideas and suggestions at a deeper level.

What is Self-Hypnosis?

Hypnosis can be done by another person, such as a hypnotherapist or hypnotist. However, self-hypnosis is when you hypnotize yourself. Hypnosis's general purpose is to bypass your conscious mind, access your subconscious, and make changes on an unconscious level.

With a self-hypnosis recording, you listen to another person and are guided through a hypnotic technique or process. Hypnosis, therefore, includes access to the subconscious. That is why we use different techniques to achieve positive changes.

The Aim of Hypnosis

Self-hypnosis often involves the use of positive suggestions. When you are relaxed, suggestions, positive ideas, or affirmations reach a much deeper level in your subconscious mind. Self-hypnosis is very useful in dealing with and changing feelings, experiences, resolving fears, accessing resources, controlling obstacles, habits, and emotions. It is often difficult to access a rational, conscious waking state. Self-hypnosis is often used to eliminate or reduce physical pain and discomfort.

Similarities Between Meditation and Self-Hypnosis

Both involve achieving an altered state of consciousness, with beta brain waves moving to the slowest alpha level.

The two have to do with a kind of dissociation. Be less aware of your physical environment and the external world and develop more internal attention. This makes you more aware of your feelings, thoughts, and emotions.

Both involve focused attention or concentration. For meditation, this can be your breath, an object, a mantra, or a recording. For self-hypnosis, these would be the suggestions from the hypnotherapist or a record of self-hypnosis.

The Difference Between Meditation and Self-Hypnosis

It looks like a straightforward question, but when you take a closer look, you see that there are so many different techniques in the two categories that make it difficult to do more than a general comparison. Although the boundary between meditation and self-hypnosis is not clearly defined, I think it is possible to distinguish it.

Hypnosis, whether self-hypnosis or administered by someone else, is actively trying to reach a part of your mind for a specific purpose. For example, if it is part of a therapy session, hypnosis can be used to explore hidden or repressed memories of the subconscious and draw the user's attention. It allows the person to overcome the problems. Hypnosis can also be used to create a positive state of mind by repeatedly citing key phrases called "affirmative statements." They can be used to help make subconscious changes by continually putting the thought into your conscious mind and waiting for it to seep through the subconscious, which is, of course, the root of the problem and the key to the solutions.

Hypnotherapy generally points to a more specific outcome. It can be weight loss, quitting smoking, phobia elimination, etc. At the beginning of a hypnotherapy session, meditation techniques can calm the conscious part of the mind. Once the chattering consciousness is silent, it can provide the subconscious mind with agreed therapeutic suggestions. Therefore, the suggestion seeks a specific therapeutic objective. Hypnotherapy focuses on a particular therapeutic outcome.

Meditation, on the other hand, is designed to help you focus your mind and center it on nothing. Yes, I said nothing because it is the most challenging thing for our conscious mind to do. Outside of periods of sleep or unconsciousness, our waking moments are filled with thoughts that we are not even aware of. When you sit down and try to clear yourself, do you realize how difficult it can be? It would help if you had specific techniques to achieve this state of mind where you don't consciously think about something in particular.

Traditional meditation is generally less structured. Meditation is often described as the absence of all thoughts. In meditation, you strive to maintain a state of calmness without consciously chattering. When conscious thoughts arise in words during meditation, you need to find a way to get rid of them. Meditating is at peace with who you are and what you do.

Meeting the expectations of others or even our expectations of ourselves causes stress. However, meditation can free your mind from all these negative thoughts and feelings and make you experience inner peace. In meditation, we want to have a calm mind, free from conscious thoughts.

A hypnosis session and a meditation session can lead you to a state of deep relaxation and guided visualization on a tranquil and calm beach. However, a hypnosis session will use this state of mind to suggest a therapeutic change in the subconscious mind. A person who meditates benefits from the tranquility and relaxation he experiences. This peace of mind can lead to enlightenment and self-improvement by improving the overall mind.

Hypnosis and meditation can cause deep relaxation. The two can claim a host of similar health benefits, but the pathways to the same destination are slightly different. In this sense, self-hypnosis is active, while meditation is passive. With self-hypnosis, you create change, while with meditation, you allow making adjustments by getting out of the way. Both are very effective for personal transformation but in very different ways. Both are relatively simple and easy to learn.

Chapter 4:
Sleep Deprivation and Weight Gain

Sleep requirements vary by age and are mainly influenced by our lifestyle and health status. Researchers cannot determine the exact amount of sleep needs for people of different ages. However, sleep needs vary from person to person, even among people of the same age group. There is a big difference between how much you need to function optimally and how much sleep you can get.

Lack of sleep occurs when a person sleeps less than necessary to be active. People vary based on the amount of sleep needed to be considered insomnia. Some people seem more resistant to the effects of sleep deprivation, while others are more vulnerable.

Scientists have linked a lack of sleep with various health problems, ranging from weight gain to a weakened immune system of all kinds.

Similar trends have also been observed in children and adolescents. Let's take a closer look at the link between sleep deprivation and weight gain:

Increased high-calorie junk food cravings

Lack of sleep causes significant changes in the way our brains respond to high-calorie foods. On days when people don't get enough sleep, high-calorie foods like chips and candies trigger stronger reactions in one part of the brain that help control motivation to eat. But at the same time, they also cause a sharp drop in activity in the frontal cortex, where consequences are evaluated, and rational decisions are made.

Disruption of carbohydrate metabolism

Lack of sleep interferes with the body's ability to metabolize carbohydrates, leading to high blood sugar levels, higher insulin levels, and accumulation of body fat. In one experiment, scientists stopped participants' sleep long enough to keep them from falling asleep soundly, but not long enough to fully wake them up. After these nights of deep sleep deprivation, the subjects' insulin sensitivity and glucose tolerance decreased by 25%.

Increased ghrelin level

Ghrelin is a hormone synthesized in the intestine and is often known as the hunger hormone. This hormone is responsible for sending signals to the brain when we are hungry. Therefore, it plays an essential role in regulating calorie intake and body fat content.

Studies show that lack of sleep increases ghrelin levels and hunger pangs in healthy, normal-weight people.

The results provide further evidence of the disruptive influence of sleep loss on the endocrine regulation of energy homeostasis, which can ultimately lead to weight gain.

Decreased metabolism at rest

Studies have shown that lack of sleep can decrease the body's metabolism at rest. It reduces the number of calories our body burns when we are completely at rest. It is influenced by age, weight, gender, muscle mass, and size. This requires additional validation, but a factor that appears to be a lack of sleep can lead to muscle loss.

Growth hormone reduction

Experts estimate that up to 75% of the human growth hormone is released during sleep. Lack of sleep reduces growth hormone levels that help regulate muscle and body fat relationships. Deep sleep is the most regenerative agent in all stages of sleep. During this phase of sleep, growth hormone is released and works to restore our body and muscles from the stress of the day.

Cortisol is increasing

Studies have also shown that lack of sleep increases cortisol levels and other inflammatory markers.

While eating well and exercising is essential to maintain a healthy weight, sleeping well is also an important part of maintaining weight. Therefore, establishing a healthy sleep pattern can help our bodies maintain a healthy weight.

Better Habits to Improve Your Sleep

Focus on now instead of thinking about tomorrow

The future will always exist, but it's not something we can control, is it? Sure, we can control most things that influence and build up to it, but we cannot control much else. Often, the things we want and hope for, or even work for, don't always reflect us along the line or according to our planned timeline. Given that we are not in control of what lies ahead, there's no need to be worried about it. Giving the wrong things too much energy without knowing where it's going will instill the idea that we are not in control of our lives. On that note, unless you're in control, can you thrive? Can you focus on the present? In essence, can you be happy or reach your goals? Thinking in this sense also translates in the context of today. Should you start on Monday—a day that is idealized as the perfect day to start something challenging, or should you just start today, the day you can control?

Jump into reality

The average human is extremely fixated on overthinking, and this is something that we don't necessarily feel like we have any control over. However, thinking about overcoming the habit of overthinking may not even feel reasonable to some. Since people who overthink are also considered much more emotional than others, hypnosis for weight loss can help individuals overcome more than just bad habits related to their diet and lifestyle. It can also help them overcome the habit of overthinking a workout, planning too much, as well as obsessing over their calorie intake. With hypnosis, you will be able to rid your mind off overthinking processes and make healthier choices, which can get you a lot farther than thinking about everything you want, or you still need to do. Finally, focusing on how your body feels when it's moving or even how it feels when it's consuming the right nutrients will trick your mind in wanting to implement change that will beneficially serve your body.

Detox your emotional state of mind

Anyone who is overweight, suffering from obesity or other eating disorders, is bound to have some type of emotional issue. Call it a psychological barrier, but it is something that holds most people back from losing weight. People don't struggle with weight loss because they are necessarily unaware of what to do. They may even know exactly what it is they must do but convince themselves that they can't get themselves to do it because of underlying emotional issues, which also translates into excuses and bad habits. Professional therapists will often prescribe their clients to feel their feelings instead of just suppressing it. Once you feel and embrace it, you can finally make use of it and let it go. This will, in return, set your body up for success as you will be able to focus on what's right for you instead of holding on to what's not.

Eat some gelatin or take glycine

It's usually best to stay clear of desserts after dinner since sweets can give you a sugar rush, making you feel pumped and more alert. But gelatin is an exception. Gelatin is made up of glycine and proline, amino acids that you might not consume in adequate amounts since they are found in the organs, bones, and fibrous tissues of animals. These amino acids are essential since they help your body boost immunity, control weight, and have proper hair, skin, and nail growth. One way to get these amino acids in your system is to consume gelatin. Aside from being a fantastic health supplement, gelatin can also help you sleep with ease. Studies show that people who eat gelatin before bedtime can sleep better and report less daytime drowsiness. Take note that we're not referring to those sugar and preservative-filled gelatin with artificial coloring. It's best to go with the unflavored ones.

Take some Magnesium

Magnesium usually gives your body an energy boost, and that same energy indirectly helps your body to be in a restful state after the boost. This is because magnesium helps your body wind down in preparation for sleep as it helps your muscles relax, giving your body a neuroprotective vibe that will not only help you fall asleep but also keep you asleep. Some people find that rubbing their bodies with magnesium lotion or oil can give them vivid dreams. Although some would feel the opposite and will have a hard time sleeping after a magnesium rub, it depends on your body system.

Read something fictional

And when I say read, I do not mean eBooks but paperbacks. Pausing to analyze some sentences or thoughts can easily make you fall asleep. Some suggest spiritual books can also help you forget about your worries as they usually aim to uplift the spirit and will put your mind to peace during bedtime.

Write a list or meditate

Your body needs to shift into sleep mode by relaxing, so it is best to spend the last hour before bedtime doing calming activities. Meditating before going to bed can also help your sleeping pattern. It is best to do the sort of mediation that allows you to relax your muscles. This type of meditation makes you tense up then relax your different muscles to promote an overall state of relaxation. Relaxing promotes better sleep as it helps with the transition between the wakefulness state and the drowsiness state. Writing a list of the things you aim to accomplish tomorrow also helps you to worry less as you have prepared a time or schedule for handling all your tasks for the next day. Some even suggest doing journaling, as it helps you release all your thoughts about the day that you just had. Clearing your mind from the stress of the day enables you to relax. This way, you won't find yourself lying awake in bed because you're worrying over something. It also helps if you keep clocks out of sight. Knowing what time, it just makes you aware that you are losing sleep, and before you know it, you're counting the hours pass by.

Chapter 5: Emotional Eating and Overeating

We have all been there! That pinch of pizza during final exams, the big cup of ice cream after a painful break, or the extra-large slice of cake after a busy day. Emotional eating as a means of reducing stress may seem like a tool for dealing with difficult emotions. So, by definition, emotional eating is normal, as most people do. Emotional eating works to manage the stress of everyday life. This eating behavior can later lead to emotional overeating or perhaps an uncontrolled eating disorder. Some emotional eaters also have to deal with anxiety, depression, or a history of traumatic experiences. One of the keys to controlling emotional eating is to incorporate awareness, or mindfulness, into eating.

Although, it is better off when people give themselves permission to eat emotionally at times, consciously, rather than guilt. Guilt creates a battle of wills to never emotionally eat again, which will likely fail and can lead to overeating. The effort to "reject, limit, and resist" does not work.

The Psychology of Emotional Eating

Emotional eating is, to some extent, physiological. When we are stressed, our bodies have an activation of the sympathetic nervous system or a "fight or flight" reaction. A rush of adrenaline is part of the fight or flight response. We need energy to "survive" stress. When we consume calories while food is metabolized, a signal is sent to the brain that the body has enough energy to run or fight, and our brain "turns off" the sympathetic (stress) response. After a few bites, our bodies feel safe and go into a state of parasympathetic nervous system, which slows us down, relaxes us, and gives us comfort. In other words, it works! But it works until it does. This is where consciousness comes into play.

Emotional eating behaviors often stem from influences from early life. Like the influence of parents and caregivers' eating habits, the foods used as a reward or punishment, programs that guide eating habits, companions, diets, and rules can also influence eating later in life. However, early and current dietary influences are rarely based on hunger.

Babies know that they can stop breastfeeding or drinking from a bottle when they are full - their bodies are tuned to the signs of hunger and satisfaction. They are the perfect conscious eaters. Later, the variety of external dietary influences disconnects the body from these intrinsic internal stimuli.

Common Causes of Emotional Eating

Stress

Have you ever noticed that stress makes you hungry?

Then you're not alone. When stress is chronic, our bodies tend to produce high levels of cortisol (the stress hormone). Cortisol evokes the need for sweet and fried foods and salty foods that give you lots of energy and joy. The higher the stress in your life, the more likely you are to turn to food for emotional relief.

Fill your emotions

Eating can be seen as a means of temporarily silencing or "filling" unpleasant feelings, such as fear, sadness, loneliness, resentment, fear, and shame. While paralyzed by food, you can avoid the difficult feelings you prefer not to have.

Boredom or feeling empty

Have you ever eaten to give yourself something to do or to fill a void in your life? You feel empty and unhappy, and food seems like a way to fill your mouth, and your time distracts you from the underlying feelings of emptiness and dissatisfaction in your life.

Childhood habits

It's normal for parents to reward their good behavior with ice cream, eat pizza if they get good grades or sweets if they are sad. Or your food can be enlivened by fond memories of grilling hamburgers with your father or eating cookies with your mother. These habits often enter adulthood.

Social influences

Eating with other people seems to be an excellent way to relieve stress, but it can also lead to overeating. It's easy to overeat simply because the food is there or because everyone eats. You can also overeat on a social occasion due to nervousness. Or maybe your family or friends encourage you to overeat.

You have probably seen yourself in at least one of the descriptions above. But if you still want to be more specific, one way to identify the patterns behind your emotional eating is to keep a journal.

When you feel compelled to overeat, take a moment to understand what is causing the urge. In this way, you will generally experience a shocking event that triggered the emotional cycle of food. Record everything in your food diary: what did you eat, how did you feel before eating, what did you feel while eating, and what did you feel after? Over time, a pattern will emerge!

Become a mindful eater

These additional tips for dealing with emotional food:

- Resist a moral value that creates embarrassment when eating: "good" versus "bad" food and "clean" versus "dirty" food.
- Ask yourself if you are starving or eating due to stress.

- Try to "control yourself". Strive to understand the different feelings of hunger during the day and meals.

- Identify the different activities that relax what you can do to avoid eating emotionally.

Using a personal "hunger indicator" can help restore body-mind communication. It internalizes the hunger signs, making it more challenging to remove external influences. The strategy is to pay more attention to how you feel and evaluate these emotions on a scale of 0 to 10. This helps the body to perceive, understand, and be more aware of the internal sensations during food.

The hunger indicator collects data and, if the experience is good, the variables (the type of food, quality, quantity, time, etc.) can be repeated. Otherwise, they can be edited and commented on mentally or in a journal. This approach to data collection also helps reduce food embarrassment, as we are less likely to overeat when we are aware of it, rather than making a mistake when eating.

Another strategy is to ask yourself if you are hungry or stressed. If you physically assess hunger before, during, and after eating, this can guide you on how much to eat and what to eat. If it is emotional, discuss step by step:

- What is the feeling?
- Where does it come from?

- Replace it with other activities that create joy and comfort.

This three-to-one relationship can help you overcome your emotional eating. Food creates joy in the brain, but many other actions can trigger pleasure. Use three more actions as a substitute to balance the pleasure of eating emotionally. This offers a break and an opportunity to control your desires.

Activities like drinking a cup of tea, having a bath, walking or listening to music, or a combination of these actions activates the parasympathetic nervous system and progressive response to relaxation and stress management.

Emotional eating is often violent and banal, as health and nutrition experts believe, this could be one of the main reasons why people are more obese than ever. We eat because we are happy or sad more than when we are starving, and the food we eat in such situations is often far from healthy. So, there is a problem because emotional eating tends to consume large amounts of unhealthy food. Obesity, diabetes, heart disease, and other health problems are the result of poor nutrition. So, it makes a lot of sense to stop eating in response to mood or feelings, and only by eating correctly can you avoid the long list of health problems.

__Moving on to an old answer: Hypnosis__

Hypnosis allows us to speak directly to the subconscious mind while avoiding the conscious mind, and relaxation techniques and specific language patterns will enable you to reprogram your mental beliefs.

If successful, hypnosis has proven to be almost a miracle cure. The list of physical and mental problems that hypnosis has been able to treat effectively is varied and almost infinite. Since your emotions are based on your thoughts and feelings, hypnosis is a logical and alternative treatment option. You speak directly to your subconscious, teaching them to avoid responding to emotions with negative feeding behaviors.

Your unconscious mind forms new habits incredibly fast, which means that hypnotherapy can quickly cure your unhealthy episodes of emotional eating when everything else you've tried has failed. Healthy hypnosis will begin with you lying down comfortably, closing your eyes and trying to eliminate thoughts and emotions from the mind.

After a few sessions, you might start to notice being more in control of your emotional reactions and dealing better with anxiety and stress; Since stress is one of the primary triggers for emotional eating, hypnosis can end it. Once and for all!

Chapter 6:
Weight Loss Hypnosis

Self-hypnosis appears to be a useful tool for losing weight. It helps you lose moderate amounts of weight steadily, resulting in safe and lasting weight loss. Combine it with exercise and get better results! Self-hypnosis has been used successfully for hundreds of years to combat various types of problems and addictions. Hypnosis was first mentioned by Avicenna, a Persian psychologist and doctor, in one of his work. Avicenna explicitly stated that another person's condition could be accepted and that he would accept the reality of hypnosis.

This does not mean that you can be forced to do things against your will. During the hypnosis session, listen to and understand each word, and if it breaks your standards, either reject the suggestion or stop hypnosis. So contrary to what you think, you can't force yourself to commit a crime in a hypnotic state. On the other hand, if you are a negative person who is capable of doing something wrong and is suggested to commit a crime during hypnosis, it is possible. This is because hypnosis is about being open to suggestions. This means that all hypnosis is self-hypnosis! The choice is yours: accept or reject an idea that has been made.

Hypnosis is beneficial in combating different types of psychological problems, addictions, and eliminating bad habits. In most hypnosis clinics, about 75% of activities involve smoking and losing weight.

You must remember that you cannot be hypnotized for doing something against your will. It is essential to have a desire to lose weight. In this way, hypnosis can be a great tool to help you achieve your goal, but contrary to what people think, it doesn't work like magic!

Also, remember that your main goal is to convince yourself to eat healthily and never overeat. It is imperative not to label what you are doing as a "diet." Most of the time, the word "diet" will make your conscious mind rebel and give you even more discomfort. Instead, be careful not to eat the entire plate. Leave a small portion of food on the plate every time you eat. Over time, you will be able to leave more and more food. With this, you send yourself a suggestion not to overeat.

Another good technique is to collect various foods responsible for the extra kilos and abstain from them for a certain period of time. Remember, what you are doing is not a diet. You are simply challenging yourself and gently stretching to do more and more.

To use self-hypnosis effectively for weight loss, prepare individual scripts that you want to hear. There are many ready-to-use here in this book. Scripts that you can use for this purpose.

The only thing that matters is your openness to suggestions, which is directly proportional to your desire to lose weight. If you are not ready to lose weight and still resist what your scenario suggests, no hypnotist can help you!

If you want to create your script, it should describe your objective behavior.

For example, I don't want to eat between meals... fatty and unhealthy food no longer appeal to me... I have full control over my eating habits...

Choose your words; Repetition is good. Your script should take at least a few minutes. Describe your desired behavior in terms that extend your current habits, but don't seem impossible to you. If it is something you cannot believe, your mind will rebel against it and have no effect. If you notice an improvement, go one step further with a new script.

Record your voice; you can save it to your iPod and listen to it several times a day. Ideally, you should listen to it when you are relaxed, but it will help you even more if you are used to listening to it, even during your daily activities.

As mentioned earlier, moderate weight loss can be achieved using only self-hypnosis. If you combine it with an increase in training, your results will be even better.

Chapter 7:
How to Prepare Yourself for Hypnosis

Hypnosis can be an effective way to lose weight, help you sleep, eliminate phobias, reduce stress, enjoy conditions, and maximize your potential. And to make these changes, you need specific words for the hypnotic state. It looks so simple, right? Well, that's because it is!

Overcoming a "serious" problem can cause a snowball effect in your mind, and you will begin to see other related issues disappear. For example, you can use hypnosis to lose weight or get fit. This, in turn, builds your confidence, and your self-esteem will also increase.

Self-hypnosis should be used not only for problems but also to simplify your life, give you more security, help you enjoy life more, improve your sport, improve your skills, or even help you learn other skills faster. Think of it as a cleansing of the mind to begin the process of creating the life you want.

It is crucial to prepare for self-hypnosis. Taking these steps should prepare the mind and body for hypnosis. I have covered some common problems that can arise, and that can induce hypnosis:

- Sit or lie down in a quiet and comfortable place.

- Dampen the lights or close the curtains.

- Make sure the tablets or phones are turned off.

- The ambient temperature should be comfortable.

- Make sure the neck is in a comfortable position. Use a pillow if necessary.

- Now close your eyes as this simplifies concentration.

- Take a few deep breaths before beginning and prepare your mind for full participation.

- Remember that hypnosis is not a passive action and requires your full participation.

For a better approach to hypnosis, don't analyze what you feel during hypnosis. If you trained in NLP or other types of mental analysis therapies, try leaving your awareness out the door so that your conscious mind remains conscious but calm during hypnosis, and your inner mind will naturally filter out what is not wanted.

If your mind is distracted during hypnosis, try to tune your thoughts to focus on the chosen induction. One way to do this is to focus your attention on the breath while continuing to listen to the induction. If you immediately deal with wandering thoughts, you will soon discover that your mind is learning a new habit, and your concentration and focus become much easier and more natural to achieve.

Chapter 8: Weight Loss Hypnosis Session

Self-Hypnosis for Weight Loss Script 1

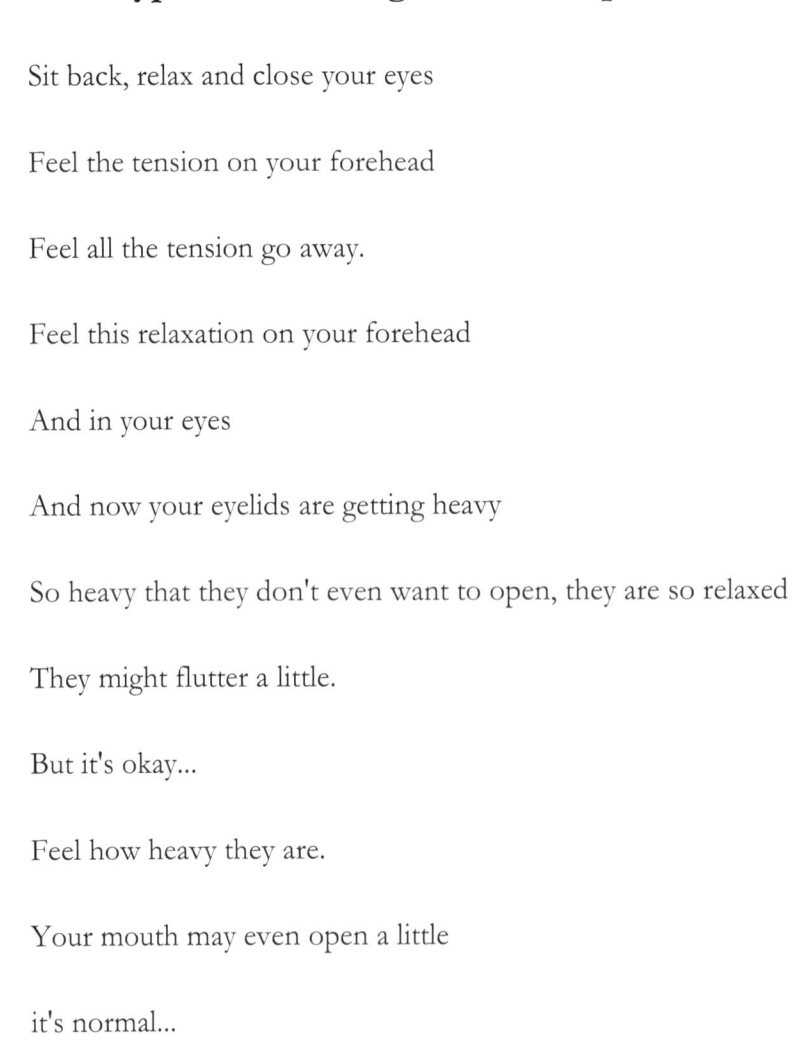

Sit back, relax and close your eyes

Feel the tension on your forehead

Feel all the tension go away.

Feel this relaxation on your forehead

And in your eyes

And now your eyelids are getting heavy

So heavy that they don't even want to open, they are so relaxed

They might flutter a little.

But it's okay...

Feel how heavy they are.

Your mouth may even open a little

it's normal...

Relax with every breath you take,

You're so relaxed now

More relaxed with each deep breath you take.

Very deep now, breathing heavier as you go deeper and deeper.

Now imagine this...

Imagine being in this beautiful and charming field

At the base of your feet, there is a wonderful walkway and brick stairs

This leads to a very safe and very relaxing forest.

These steps will take you to a very deep state of deep hypnosis.

Get these steps together now.

While counting down from 10 to 0

Each problem will take you deeper and deeper.

That's right, very good; it's going very well now.

10: take that first step down

9: getting deeper

8: now down

7: even deeper

6: so wonderfully relaxed

5: Deeper and deeper

4: you are now entering a state of deep and deep hypnosis

3: deepen

2: so relaxed that you can even move around, feeling very, very comfortable. More comfortable than ever, never felt before

1: you will enter this beautiful place of peace and tranquility called deep and deep hypnosis.

0: continues to go deeper and deeper, so calm and so relaxed; Continue to relax now, breathing easily and listening to light music as you go further and further.

Imagine a door,

right in front of you

It has a positive sign on the door.

the positive sign must mean that you enter;

When you open the door, you see five steps;

Descending to a room full of dials and meters on all the walls.

Go down those steps

Please note that all counters and dials seem to continue indefinitely.

There are so many meters and dials

But when you look at them, you notice that they are individually labeled.

A meter is labeled "metabolism."

The other is labeled "cholesterol."

Another is labeled "blood pressure."

And another labeled "body fat and weight."

And while you look at millions and millions of meters and quadrants,

You will realize that you are in the control room of your mind

Sitting in the center of this control room is a book called "perfect health."

It has your name in the book.

Go to that book

Take a look inside

Scroll through the words

Begin to see that each page has an image of each quadrant and a configuration in the quadrant;

What represents perfect health for you.

Start scrolling through the pages

As you scroll through the book, you see a mirror in the corner of the room.

You approach the mirror

While you look at yourself in this mirror

Imagine the mirror showing all the different angles

In this mirror, you see a perfect reflection of you with the correct weight and size you want to be.

Look at you from all angles

With all the curves in the right places

Your clothes adapt perfectly to your body.

As you look at the true beauty of your reflection,

Listen to your reflection by giving them these suggestions:

From now on I will chew my food longer and slower

From now on, when I sit down to eat;

I will measure my hunger level on a scale of one to ten.

Zero is starving and ten are so full that I can't eat another bite.

From now on, I will stop eating at 6 or 7.

Now I want to eat a fresh and healthy source of vegetables.

Keep in mind that your reflection reaches out to touch yours,

When his hands come in contact, you feel an unconditional source of love from your unconscious reflection.

Feel the intimate source of love pouring into your heart

And now you see your reflection reaching out your hand

When you reach out to take your reflection;

Step forward in your reflection as you become your reflection.

Feel how nice it is to become your reflection

Come out of the mirror into a new life of health and vitality.

Go back to your perfect health control room

Allow yourself to make safe and moderate adjustments.

Start drawing your attention to the sensations inside your body

As you feel, you begin to correct.

That's right...

Feel the sensations

Feel the perfect weight you want

As your body begins to move towards perfect size

Achieving your desired weight

I will count from 1 to 5 and by doing so, you will wake up.

With every count, you'll make sure these suggestions are deep in your unconscious mind:

1: see yourself the size and shape you want to be, you deserve to be.

2: feel wonderful about yourself, finally knowing that you are in control

3: you want healthy foods to help you weigh your ideal weight

4: ready now to do whatever it takes to accomplish this and

5: eyes open, fully awake, bright and alert, now fully awake.

That's right...

Self-Hypnosis for Weight Loss Script 2

Please make yourself comfortable

Settle in...

Don't worry about how deeply you relax you are and go into a trance

You don't even have to try.

Just listen...

Take a deep breath

and other

Keep noticing your slow, steady breathing

Pay close attention to the feeling that the chest rises and falls

Feel that positive air pressure

With the breath coming

As you release the air

You can even imagine that the air is safe,

Healing color when it enters and leaves your body

It also guides you to a deeply relaxed state

Now you are relaxed...

Time to treat the part of you that doesn't want to lose weight.

Part of you can rebel against your target

That's it...

This part of you that doesn't want to lose weight

Now you can face that part of you

Not as an enemy or a victim.

But as a long-lost friend

This part of you that is hurt

Rejected by others

Rejected by you

And now is the time to heal.

Now is the time to make peace inside of you

Now you have the opportunity to reconcile

Slowly, consistently, and successfully reach your ideal weight

Let this happen...

Let these words sink in as you say you hear them:

I'm sorry you're hurt.

You have been hurt by others.

You have been ignored by me.

It's time to heal...

I would like you to feel loved.

Let's work together

Let's end this war

We can make peace. It depends on us.

Imagine making peace with yourself now.

And feel the healing energy going through your body.

By pooling their strengths and resources,

Heal your weaknesses and close the gap that has been in your soul,

It prevents you from fully embracing your healthiest sense of self.

You

are a genuine human being

With all your strengths available to all parts of yourself.

Be proud of yourself

Show yourself in your thoughts and feelings.

You'll soon discover all the parts of yourself that align with your healthiest sense of self

Physically, mentally, emotionally, and spiritually.

Healthy food will taste wonderful.

Unhealthy food will taste fake, empty, and lifeless.

You will be motivated to move your body.

Invites a vibrant feeling of general well-being and fitness.

Go ahead and make peace on the inside

Stay strong on the outside.

Begin to see weight loss come naturally.

Allow what you learned in this session to be integrated into your being

And when you choose to imagine yourself in front of a mirror.

Imagine that you are in your favorite outfit.

With the exact weight you want

Feel relaxed, awake and hopeful.

Imagine that your body weight begins to move towards the desired weight.

Now take your time...

With every count, you'll make sure these suggestions sink deep in your unconscious mind:

1: see yourself the size and shape you want to be, you deserve to be.

2: feel wonderful about yourself, finally knowing that you are in control

3: you want healthy foods to help you weigh your ideal weight

4: ready now to do whatever it takes to accomplish this

5: eyes open, fully awake, bright and alert, now fully awake.

That right...

Self-Hypnosis for Weight Loss Script 3

Please make yourself comfortable

Take a deep breath

Relaxing with every breath

You're so relaxed now

Keep noticing your slow, steady breathing...

Pay close attention to the feeling that the chest rises and falls

With the breath coming

Feel that positive air pressure

Just relax...

Feel that your eyelids are becoming heavy

So heavy that they don't even want to open

But it's okay...

Now to decide the time to lose weight

Create an image in your mind of your future self at your ideal weight on that date.

I want you to see exactly how you will look.

See how happy you will be.

And imagine how happy you will feel.

Make the image big and bright.

You can feel that smile grow as you easily imagine

Easily reach your goal

See how compelling that image is to you.

Now create a new image in your mind halfway to your goal.

Imagine how happy you will feel, knowing that you are halfway to your goal.

Look how good you are.

See how much has improved since today.

And I want you to imagine waking up tomorrow morning

Full of energy, knowing that you are on the way to achieving your goal,

Knowing that the more you see your end goal, the easier it will be

Go effortlessly and get exactly what you want.

Now I want your unconscious to make a change

Imagine your goal and motivate yourself even more

Understand what it means to you now.

Learn to enjoy exercise.

Look forward to getting around every day!

Eliminate you're eating compulsions

Eat healthily

Change your daily eating habits

Feel the sensations

Feel the perfect weight you want

Feel your body weight begin to move towards perfect size

Achieve the desired weight

I will count from 1 to 5 and by doing so, you will wake up.

With every count, you'll make sure these suggestions are deep in your unconscious mind:

1: see yourself the size and shape you want to be, you deserve to be.

2: feel wonderful about yourself, finally knowing that you are in control

3: you want healthy foods to help you weigh your ideal weight

4: ready now to do whatever it takes to accomplish this and

5: eyes open, fully awake, bright and alert, now fully awake. Straight.

Meditation for Weight Loss

Take a comfortable position.

Close your eyes when you start to relax.

Take a deep breath; now exhale, completely emptying your lungs.

And one more time. Take a deep breath, never strain or rush.

Breathe vigorously; exhale the tension.

Continue to breathe this way to relax.

Take a deep breath.

Allow your breathing to discover its natural and unhurried rhythm.

And as ideas enter your mind, allow them to float without attachment.

Now say to yourself:

I would like to eat smaller and smaller amounts of food.

I'll remember that filling feeling; I get after eating too much on thanksgiving

I don't like that filling feeling.

I am enjoying my new way of eating. Very slowly, always placing my cutlery between the bites and thinking only of the bite that is in my mouth

I will always leave food on my plate. Much, much better not eating it all then eating too much.

I will like it much more. My taste buds become more sensitive. And I get much more satisfaction with every bite than I eat

Fattening and sweet foods repel me. It always reminds me of a plate of granulated sugar with thick sticky molasses poured over it.

I will reduce excess weight little by little, day by day, week by week.

Until I reach my weight goal of [x]. And I know that I will feel more energetic.

And therefore, I will continue my exercise.

The more I train, the better I feel and the better I feel, the more I train.

I am better and I feel better.

My clothes are coming off. I feel good about myself.

I have more confidence. I smile more easily. Because I know that I will win...

(PAUSE)

Remember that you can return to this place whenever you want.

For a moment, remind yourself of the sense of peace that is yours.

Open your eyes

Feel the goodness of meditation for a few moments.

(PAUSE)

That's right...

Chapter 9:
Deep Sleep Hypnosis

What is Deep Sleep Hypnosis?

Hypnosis is considered to be an excellent way to treat sleeping disorders. With hypnosis for deep sleep, a person can relax and regulate the mind to get a good and restoring sleep. It allows us to touch our subconscious mind and discover the source of our fear and hesitation. This therapy guides our minds to relieve our worries, to relax, and concentrate on this calm state.

Sleep hypnosis turns sleeping disorders into a healthy pattern of sleep. This method stimulates our subconscious into a deep state of rest and sleep, thus keeping a person sufficiently energetic in the morning. We don't have to take drugs such as tablets or drinks to sleep well. We only have to calm our minds and bodies and rejuvenate ourselves with our well-deserved rest. This treatment can help us to sleep like a baby.

During deep sleep, glucose metabolism in the brain increases, which is essential for short-term and long-term memory as well as for overall learning. It is during the deep sleep phase when the pituitary gland in the brain secretes vital hormones, including the human growth hormone, which is crucial for the growth and development of the body.

The lack of sufficient amounts of deep sleep can cause a lot of problems. It is during this phase of sleep when the information accumulated through the day is processed. When deep sleep is not enough, the brain cannot convert and store this information to your memory.

The lack of quality sleep, which is essentially embedded in your deep sleep phase, is also connected to other health disorders like heart disease, Alzheimer's disease, stroke, and diabetes. The deep sleep stage is also associated with certain sleep-related disorders like night terrors, sleepwalking, sleep eating, and bedwetting.

In truth, deep sleep is not a specific requirement. However, younger people need it more than older people because of the growth hormone that is released during that time, which is vital for growth and development. While older people also need some amount of deep sleep, not getting enough of it, does not necessarily translate to having a sleep disorder

Deep Sleep for Weight Loss

It is without a doubt that sleep quality has a direct influence on our body weight. However, most people are yet to discover the secret to a good night's sleep? If you want more rest, "deep sleep hypnosis" can be very useful.

Deep sleep hypnosis is meant to help us:

- Sleep faster.
- To ensures restful sleep.

Sleep quality is often the last place most people look at when they are frustrated with health conditions. But then sleeping is a fundamental part of a healthy life. Poor sleep quality takes away energy, strength, and appearance. It prevents the mind and body from effectively controlling hunger, weight, and cravings.

If a good night's sleep doesn't seem like enough motivation to make sleep quality a priority, keep in mind that it will help you on your journey to weight loss.

If restless sleep is a health killer, then think about what restful sleep can do for your entire being. Restful sleep acts as a bath at the end of the day.

Instead of letting stress build-up and continue through the night, you can press the refresh button in a deep sleep, waking up mentally and physically during the day.

Sleep quality is more than a mathematical equation.

It's not enough to keep your eyes closed and lie down for 7-8 hours. Deep sleep hypnosis teaches the mind and body to transform these 7-8 hours into deep, regenerative sleep. Too often, we miss the benefits of a good night's sleep, and mornings always seem to come too early. But imagine being excited when your alarm rings, feeling refreshed and ready to go.

It is the power of deep sleep, and it is what you should have every night.

Consider deep sleep hypnosis as a powerful tool to access your subconscious and connect with you and your needs. Think of it as a guided meditation. Deep sleep hypnosis gives you the power to train your mind on deep sleep, which your body needs to lose weight.

Chapter 10:
How to Prepare Yourself to Sleep Hypnosis

Self-hypnotization can do wonders for your health and may also sound far too good to be true. However, many experts believe that changing our thought processes can lead to a much better state of health and quality of life.

To prepare yourself for this practice, you should:

Implement Powerful Breathing Techniques

Integrating powerful breathing, including diaphragmatic breathing, is terrific for amplifying your focus. When we focus on deep or controlled breath, both our minds and bodies enter a state of being calm, allowing us to feel like we are in control. This also opens the door to feeling happier, allowing us to implement more positive habits and experiences into our days, rather than just going through a motion rut. Focusing on diaphragmatic breathing causes you to breathe deeply, which, when you breathe out, tightens and flattens your stomach. It relaxes your body and also creates the idea of visualization that you can indeed have a flat stomach.

Apart from diaphragmatic breathing, you should also try out Buteyko breathing. This type of breathing involves breathing small quantities of fresh air in and out of your nose, which reduces the total amount of oxygen you use. Given that most individuals over-breathe, they can't control their bodies when they are stressed. It contributes to lousy digestion, inadequate sleeping patterns, and many other negative habits that support weight gain. Implementing this breathing technique can solve one issue you struggle with but can translate into solving countless other problems you face. It will also reduce anxiety and place you in a more mindful state of living.

What to Do Before Bedtime

A comfortable and quiet sleeping area is critical for a good night's rest. A noisy, bright room that is either too hot or cold is not conducive to sleep. If you live in a noisy neighborhood, using earplugs or a sound machine is a good idea to keep out the disturbances from outside.

Also, make sure your room is cool. You can either keep a window open or use a fan. An eye mask or blackout curtains can help keep out all kinds of bright lights streaming in through the windows.

Make sure your pillow and mattress are comfortable. Try out different mattresses and pillows and identify one that works best for you.

Heat is known to promote deep sleep. Therefore, it might be a great idea to take a hot bath before bedtime to improve your sleep quality. Low-carb diets and certain antidepressants are also known to promote sleep, although research work in this realm is still needed for a clearer understanding.

Avoid caffeine and other decaffeinated drinks as your bedtime approaches. Water is your best bet to quench thirst. Avoid alcohol and nicotine also before bedtime as it hampers sleep quality.

Do not eat heavy meals for dinner, and also make sure you eat early. Rich, heavy foods should be entirely avoided at least a couple of hours before your bedtime. Acidic or spicy foods can give you stomach problems as well as heartburns.

Avoid all kinds of stimulating activity before your bedtime. For example, don't check out social media messages, have discussions and arguments with your partner or family member, or try catching up on work. Keep all these activities for the morning and get into bed at your scheduled time.

Loud noises and bright lights should be banished from your bedroom. Also, switch off electronic devices, including TV, mobiles, and the computers at least an hour before your bedtime. The blue light emitted by electronic devices disrupts the production of melatonin, an essential hormone for sleep, in your body.

Avoid drinking too much liquid before bedtime. Getting up for frequent toilet visits is likely to hamper the quality of your sleep. Stop drinking anything at least an hour before bedtime, which is a great way to limit bathroom visits at night.

Right Time to Go to Bed

Keep a regular sleep schedule - Ensure you align your life with your biological clock. Keep a proper time to sleep and wake up. This regular sleeping schedule should be maintained on weekends too. Sometimes, it is reasonable to want to sleep in late because you are tired. Try and avoid falling for this trap because your sleep rhythm is likely to get disturbed. Instead, wake up at the same time each day, even if you are feeling tired. This approach will help you regain your regular sleeping rhythm.

Have a regular sleep schedule, and make sure you go to bed and wake up at the same time each day.

The Environment

Be sure to darken your room until it is pitch-black. When you eliminate all sources of light in your bedroom, your body system automatically shuts down in the darkness. Even the light emitting from the hallway under your doors is enough to distract you from sleeping. Try placing some rags or a thick mat under your door for total darkness. Use blinds on your windows instead of curtains so that you can block out light from streaming in your bedroom through your windows easily. Remember that the tiniest bit of light—even the soft glow from your alarm clock—can interfere with your sleep. You can also simply use an eye mask to trick your brain that you are in total darkness if you have family members or roommates who are not ready to turn off all the lights yet in your home.

Make sure that there are absolutely no distractions that can prevent you from making the most out of this hypnosis. Play the sounds that you find comforting as well, preferably the ones with isochoric tones to remain focused. Have you noticed that it's easier to sleep or take a nap when it's raining? This is because the sound of falling rain is calming and relaxing. You can listen to nature sounds such as rain, running water, birds tweeting, the sounds of a forest or an ocean while going to sleep. Listening to such tracks can help you ease up and relax, and before you know it, you'd be drifting off to dreamland.

If you have an essential oil diffuser, you should set it up before lying down as well. In case you do not own one, then apply the essential or aromatic oil of your choice on your temples or wrists. Nevertheless, you can do away without such oils, too. They are merely optional tools that may help you ascertain that you are ready to start the hypnosis before bed and that you are well-prepared to do it. Once all of that is done, the next thing that you want to do is make sure that you end up in a comfortable position. This way, you can genuinely get into a state of relaxation so that you will be able to get into a deep sleep.

The Right Posture

What is the best position/posture to sleep? Well, that is going to be up to what is the most comfortable pose for you when it comes to slumbering in bed. Anyone who is going to be doing this deep-sleep meditation needs to get into the most comfortable position. Think of it as if you are getting ready to snooze for the night.

Being in a position that is not going to bring you the most comfort will defeat the purpose of the guide and will not allow you to meditate effectively.

Chapter 11:
Meditation to Calm an Overactive Mind

Breathe deeply three times and purge your body of stress. As you breathe in each time, hold your breath to the count of four and release slowly.

Breathe in.

Release.

Breathe in.

Release.

Breathe in.

Release.

Your objective today is to teach yourself how to fall asleep and to relax. Over time, you may have forgotten how to fall asleep and how to release the stronghold you have on your unconsciousness so that you can allow your mind to recharge.

Start by asking yourself why you are having such a difficult time falling asleep.

Is there a specific thought that is worrying you?

Is there a list of things that you need to get done?

Is there a prospective outcome that you are nervous about?

Whatever it is that is keeping your mind constantly engaged, I want you to take a minute and truly focus on it.

Ask yourself if there is anything for you to do now, in this moment.

Breathe in.

Release.

You'll notice that, despite the fact that there is nothing to do at this moment, your consciousness is finding it difficult to release this particular thought.

Empty your mind's eye and open a blank sheet of paper. Mentally type up the problems and the fears that you have, which are constantly breaking through your consciousness. Here, you are downloading your worries and your fears so that they are no longer grasping on to your mind.

Once you are done, close the document, and refresh your mind.

You are clear.

You are unburdened.

You are light.

Your thoughts and worries are there and will remain there for you to return to tomorrow. For now, you are meant to focus only on your own consciousness.

Breathe in.

Release.

Breathe in.

Release.

Breathe in.

Release.

Today, you choose to be unburdened and, in turn, you feel that choice free you of the heavy weight that is upon your shoulders.

Remember that today, you are free, you are not tied down, and you are not fettered.

You have the ability to feel the tension in your neck and shoulders slowly release as you allow yourself to sink comfortably into the arms of relaxation.

Feel relaxation sink deeper into your bones and radiate from your spine and ribs all the way down to your toes. Every part of your body is releasing energy, and as you slowly continue to release it, you are allowing the comfortable cradle of sleep to rock you into a melodic lull.

Repeat the following with your soul: 'Today, I choose relax. My goal today is to release the tension from my body and to free myself from all forms of awareness.'

Breathe deeply to the count of four, and as you breathe out, allow the weight of your consciousness to lower your eyelids.

You are falling deeper and deeper into your unconsciousness.

Breathe in.

Release.

Breathe in.

Release.

Breathe in.

Release.

Chapter 12: Meditations for Relaxation and Self-Image

The following two scripts are intended to work together. While the first one is designed to lead you into a deep relaxation state, the second to focus on your self-image. Since the own self-image is a belief implanted in our deep subconscious, a state of deep relaxation will allow you to manipulate it more effectively. However, if you are confident with relaxation techniques and you know how to relax rapidly, you can skip the first script and jump directly to the second one.

Script 1

To get into this meditation, make sure that you are keeping your eyes closed and focused only on falling asleep. For the remainder of the meditation, we are going to use "I" statements. Remember to think of these thoughts as they come into your mind as if they were your own. As we count down from ten, make sure to focus on your breathing, and making your body as relaxed as possible.

Ten, nine, eight, seven, six, five, four, three, two, one.

I can feel my body get lighter and lighter as I relax my muscles and melt into the bed. I can tell that my body is tired and needs to be relaxed at this point. It is important that I nestle myself into bed so that I can better get the rest I need to start the day off tomorrow.

As I start to become more and more relaxed, I feel like my bed is turning into a cloud. Each breath I let out, I feel myself relaxing more and more. The air that I breathe in is energy that's going to help me feel even more relaxed.

As I breathe in, I feel all of the things that happened to me today, but as I breathe out, I let these thoughts go and pay no more attention to them. As I'm breathing in, I accept all that has happened to me today, and as I breathe out, I let go, knowing that holding onto it is only going to cause me more stress.

With every breath that I let out, I feel lighter and lighter. Each time I let the breath out, I feel like I'm sinking deeper into the clouds. I know now that I do not have to carry all of the weight with me that I have been feeling throughout the day.

I can become more and more relaxed, letting myself float and become lighter and lighter. I am drifting away from my bed now, being lifted away like a big fluffy cloud. I am not afraid of anything that I might be leaving behind. I know that it is okay to drift up and away, into the sky and looking down below me.

I am drifting from all of my responsibilities. I do not have to take care of them now. They'll be there when I get back. Right now, I only need to focus on drifting into the sky and becoming relaxed. The only thing that I need to think about is becoming more tired, feeling the fluffy cloud around me that keeps me nice and cozy.

Worrying about the things that I have to do later is not going to help me feel any better now.

I do not need to really worry about this, however. It is not a pressing issue. I might not be asleep, but at least I am resting my body.

As I look down, I see all of the people that aren't yet resting theirs. They could be in bed, but they chose to be out late. They could be drifting in the clouds, sleepy like me, but instead they are staying awake, making it harder for themselves to think and function throughout the day tomorrow.

I am taking care of my health. I am looking out for myself tomorrow. By making sure that I am focused on relaxing and falling asleep, I am ensuring that tomorrow will be an easy day for me. Tomorrow I will be relaxed, because I'm making sure that I'm tired now.

Sometimes, it is hard for me to fall asleep because I do not spend enough time winding down. It can take a little longer to get fully relaxed, and I need to remember that as I'm trying to fall asleep. It will be easier for me now to fall asleep because I am paying special attention to really winding down.

I can feel my body becoming more and more relaxed as I regulate my breathing.

As I am floating above on my fluffy cloud, I can see the wind ripple through the tree leaves. I can feel that air blow through my hair, traveling gently into my lungs. As I take a big deep breath in, I can feel how this air fills me with so much relaxation. I let the wind out slowly, and I become one with the world around me. Though not everyone is asleep, I can still feel the peace and serenity that exists all throughout this beautiful sky.

As I continue to let the air enter and exit my body, I get higher and higher. Before I know it, I can see the clouds around me, making pure gray surroundings. Some stars are still twinkling through the clouds, and I can see the black night sky behind them. As I look down, I see less and less as I become enveloped within the cloud.

Where I am now, I can no longer see the cloud that I'm actually lying on. Where my original cloud starts and stops is no longer easily identifiable. I have become one with all of the clouds at this point.

I am still floating, not worried about what's going on below me.

There is nothing around, and I feel that relaxation in every part of my body. It has never been easier than it is now to completely relax and focus only on this moment.

I can twist and move my body a bit and that will change where and how I am traveling throughout the sky. I have no plan for where I'm going, however. It doesn't really matter if I go forward, backward, left or right. The only thing I care about is feeling every last ounce of my body relax.

It is not until now, when I'm up in the clouds, that I really realize just how much tension I carry throughout my body.

Now that I am here, nowhere, nothing around me but clouds, I realize that I can feel like this all the time.

Never before have I been so tired, and now I am ultimately relaxed so I can get a full and deep night's sleep.

The more that I practice going up into the clouds like this, the easier it will be to fall asleep on a regular basis. I can do this when I'm napping, if I wake up in the middle of the night, or simply when I initially try to fall asleep.

If I want to ensure that I can fall asleep easily and stay asleep, I need to relax my entire body.

The cloud is starting to drift down now, and I understand what it means to completely let go of everything that I am feeling and allow myself to become more rested.

The cloud is passing over the streets now, and I can see that so many people are focused on getting back into bed. My cloud is moving towards my house, doing all the work so that I can remain as still and calm as possible. I do not have to worry about doing anything other than becoming entirely asleep.

My cloud gently puts me back into my bed. I can feel the warm blankets around me and the soft mattress beneath me. Everything that I experienced throughout the day is over now, and I do not have to worry about doing anything other than drifting away. Everything that stressed me out is over, and what waits tomorrow is beyond anything I can predict.

I can still feel my eyes become heavier; my breathing slower. When I reach one, I will be almost all the way asleep.

Ten, nine, eight, seven, six, five, four, three, two, one.

Script 2

Now that you are completely relaxed, I want you to take note of how you are feeling as a whole. How are you doing at this moment? How does your body feel?

Take a few moments and scan your body. There is no need to judge yourself right now. All I want you to do is notice is how your body is feeling from your head to your toes.

Scan through your body from your feet…to your ankles…all the way up your legs…and into your hips. At your own pace, scan your body through your stomach, chest, hands, shoulders, neck, head, and face.

As you focus on your body, notice how it begins to relax with no conscious effort. As you scan your body, feel as the muscles become looser and less tense on their own. All you need to do is lay quiet and remain relaxed. You feel happy that this is happening naturally. With each passing moment, your body falls more relaxed, even more, ready to fall asleep.

Now that you are feeling more relaxed, I want to talk about your body image. Many of us move through the day, uncomfortable, simply because we are not happy with ourselves and the way we look. But what is body image? Are you thinking about what your body looks like? Perhaps you are thinking about the ideas you have about your body. How are you feeling about your physical self at this moment? What does body image mean to you?

Inhale…and exhale…

As you continue to focus on your breath, I invite you to take a few moments to consider the thoughts and ideas you have about your body. How do these thoughts make you feel as you scan over your own body image? For some, you may feel comfortable and content. For others, you are unhappy, unaccepting, or dissatisfied. Perhaps, there is a combination depending on how kind you are to yourself. However, you feel, accept the emotions you are feeling at this moment.

Stay with me for a moment. I invite you to ponder how it would feel to accept your body the way it is? How would it feel to be okay with your physical self? Take a few moments now to breathe, and picture in detail how this would feel.

Breathe in…and breathe out…wonderful.

Now, try to think of a moment in your life when you accepted your physical self. Whether it be your whole self or a part of yourself that you really enjoy, think of a moment.

Which part of your body do you accept?

Imagine now, how it would feel to accept your whole body as opposed to thinking of yourself as a collection of separate parts. If you are beginning to feel stressed out over these thoughts, allow us to take a few steps back to return to relaxation.

Notice certain parts tensing up at this moment. Make a note of these locations and focus positive energy to return these body parts to total relaxation. Inhale…and exhale…you are safe and loved at this moment. You are calm and relaxed…inhale…and exhale…

When you return to a state of total relaxation and calm, I invite you to repeat the following body image affirmations after me. If you don't feel like repeating these, try to listen and relax as I speak. As you work on a positive body image, you may feel less stressed throughout the day. When we love ourselves, it grants us the ability to spread that love to others. Perhaps if you loved yourself more, you would take the time to release stress and enjoy a peaceful night's rest. Who knows, perhaps your body image has been bringing you down more than you ever imagined.

When you are ready, repeat after me. Each affirmation I am about to say is entirely true. Even if you don't believe it, you will work through your negative thoughts until you believe them to be so. Let's begin.

I am perfect the way I am.

(Pause)

I choose to accept the way I am.

(Pause)

My body is acceptable the way it is at this moment.

(Pause)

I choose to accept the body I am in.

(Pause)

I am a wonderful person as a whole.

(Pause)

There is no reason to be perfect.

(Pause)

I have imperfections, and that is okay.

(Pause)

I love the person that I am.

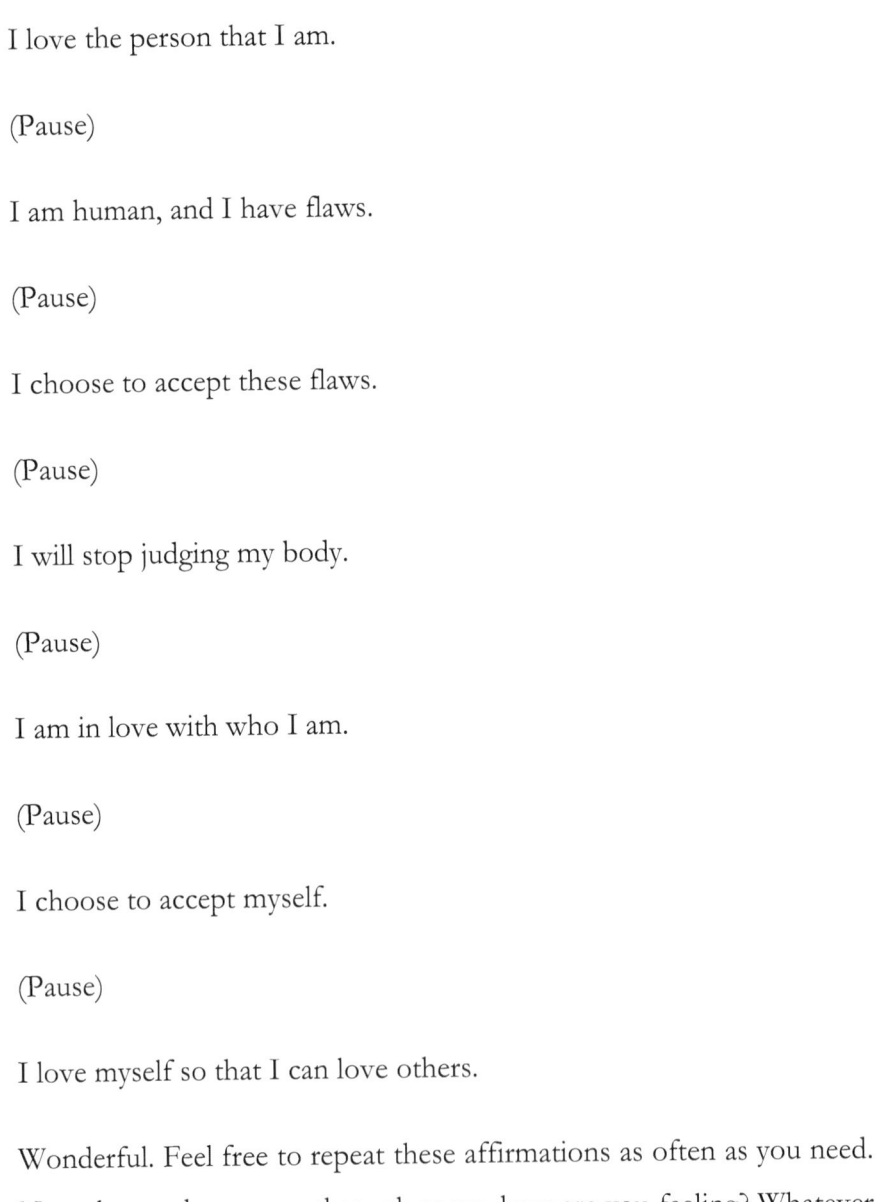

(Pause)

I am human, and I have flaws.

(Pause)

I choose to accept these flaws.

(Pause)

I will stop judging my body.

(Pause)

I am in love with who I am.

(Pause)

I choose to accept myself.

(Pause)

I love myself so that I can love others.

Wonderful. Feel free to repeat these affirmations as often as you need. Now that we have gone through some, how are you feeling? Whatever you are feeling at this moment is perfectly acceptable. Perhaps you believe every word I have told you, and perhaps you don't. As you practice positive body image more, you may find yourself becoming less stressed and much happier.

Inhale…and two…and three…and four…and pause…two…three…and exhale…two…three…four…five…

You are doing wonderfully. In a few moments, we will be moving onto exercises so you can fall asleep. Before we get there, I want you to turn your focus inward. Take a deep, truthful look inside to find your authentic self.

As you do this, begin to reflect on your values. What is important to you? What do you value most in life? Why is it that you chose this audio to help release stress so that you can sleep better at night? For the next few moments, I invite you to focus on your breath and ask yourself these very important questions.

(Pause)

Breathe in…breathe out…

What is left when you strip all of these problems away? This person is who you are at the core. All of your character traits and personality makes you who you are, and that is all you can ask of yourself. You work hard. You are a committed person. You are in love with your life.

With all of these positive changes you have made in just one night, it is time to put your mind to rest. You have done a wonderful job of working on your well-being. At this moment, you are feeling calm and relaxed. You have let go of your worries, explored your true self, and found your authentic core. When you are ready, take a deep breath in and let it go.

At this moment, you should feel completely calm and at peace. Your body begins to gently tell you that it is time to fall asleep. In the next few moments, we will begin to place your mind and soul at rest. You will sleep peacefully and deep through the night. In the morning, you will awaken feeling calm and well rested at the time you need to wake up.

Chapter 13: Deep Sleep Hypnosis

In the previous chapter, we went through meditation to calm our mind. This state of peace is essential to prepare further actions. Whether we want to work on ourselves or to go deeper in the relaxation to induce mindfulness, or to sleep better, we have to learn how to achieve our inner peace.

Now it's time to enjoy a good night's sleep, and deep sleep hypnosis is a powerful tool to make the best of our relaxing time. By lengthening the period in which our mind rests in the state of deep sleep, we can boost the healing and restoring functions that sleep has over our body, brain...and weight!

Script 1

I want you to start in the most comfortable position possible. Switch the light off and become aware of the background music in this session. Isn't it soothing? Allow your thoughts to flow with the calm rhythm of the sound you hear. As you fade the sound of the music just slightly, you grab onto the sound of my voice. Listen to the sound of my voice and the background music in harmonious balance. I want you to close your eyes. Your eyes are feeling droopy now. You have had a long day and your eyes are allowed to feel heavy. Keep your eyes closed and use your sense of hearing to follow my suggestions. You feel a deepening trust in my instructions with every word I speak. Allow my suggestions to flow through your mind, bringing more comfort with each moment.

You are going to focus on your breathing now. I want gentle inhales and exhales. Keep a consistent rhythm with each breath you take. Feel your body soften further with each exhale. Stop thinking about the thing that just crossed your mind and come back to me. I want you to feel a small wave of guilt for allowing your mind to wander. Now start your breathing over again. Small, shallow breaths—gently in and gently out. Your breathing to slow your heartbeat, one breath at a time. Your eyes are feeling more and more drowsy with each beat of your heart. Your mind refuses to shut down and you don't know why. Shift your focus back to your breathing now and follow the air as it flows into your body. You can feel your body rise and fall as you inhale and follow the flow of air as it exits your body. You are becoming more confident in this session.

Now I want you to focus on your breathing again. Make sure it remains steady. Feel your body conform to each inhale and exhale. Your arms are too relaxed and you don't feel the need to touch your body to feel this. You are in an unfamiliar state of mind now. You have become one with your subconscious mind. You feel a deeper need to trust the sound of my voice now as the time draws nearer. All doubts have swiftly removed themselves. It's just you and my voice now.

Script 2

I want you to get comfortable. Because you are trying to achieve deep sleep, you should be lying down, your head resting on your most comfortable pillow, and warmed by your softest blanket. Lie back and let your shoulders go slack, relaxing against the cushion of your bed. Gently close your eyes and release all the tension from your muscles. Release the tension in your arms, then your legs. Let go of the tension in your chest and in your back. All of the muscles in your body begin to feel looser and looser and your body is feeling light.

Focus your attention on your toes. Softly wiggle all ten toes once, and then again. Feel the energy released from your movement and the stillness that follows. Your toes are now ready for sleep.

Next, tighten the muscles in your calves and hold for one, two, three seconds. Now release the muscles. Tighten them again for one, two, three seconds. Now release. The excess energy that keeps you up at night has been expelled from your calves. Your calves are now ready for sleep.

Next, squeeze your thigh muscles and hold for one, two, three seconds. Now release. The tension that was once stored there has been released. Your thighs are now ready for sleep. Feel the lightness that has cloaked your legs. Your legs feel weightless as if they could float up to the ceiling.

Focus your attention on your buttocks. Tighten your muscles in buttocks for one, two, three seconds. Now release the muscles. The tightness in your buttocks and lower back has been relieved. Your buttocks and lower back are now ready for sleep.

Focus your attention on your abdomen. Squeeze your abdominal muscles for one, two, three seconds. Now release. The anxiety that has been stored up and deterring sleep has been released. Your abdomen is now ready for sleep.

Concentrate on your chest. Tighten the muscles in your chest for one, two, three seconds. Now release. The sadness that has been weighing on you and preventing your mind from resting has been expelled. Your chest is now ready for sleep.

Direct your attention now to your shoulders. Tighten the muscles in your shoulder for one, two, three seconds. Now release. The stress that has been building in the deep tissue of your shoulders has now been dissolved. Your shoulders are now ready for sleep.

Focus your attention on your neck. Gently tighten the muscles and hold for one, two, three seconds. Now release. Gently tighten the muscles in your jaw and hold for one, two, three seconds. Now release. Gently tighten the muscles in your mouth and hold for one, two, three seconds. Now release. Gently squeeze your eyelids tighter for one, two, three seconds. Now release. The tension that was held in your face has now been released.

Imagine that you are a leaf on a tree. You are connected to a giant colony of other leaves attached to a branch. That branch is attached to a trunk.

You are a part of a busy, ever rustling tree. However, you want to be still. You need to rest. You need to separate yourself from the busyness of your world. You decide that you will depart your branch and you begin to float. Slowly, as if gravity has slowed your fall, you twirl and roll in the breeze. You are peacefully drifting further and further, reassured that you are safe.

Instead of the ground, you see that there is a quiet pond below your tree and soon you will touch the surface. As you float towards it, you notice its stillness. There are no ripples or disturbances. The surface is smooth and clear; it is as reflective as a mirror. As you reach the water, you greet the surface with a delicate kiss.

You send gentle, peaceful ripples from your contact. Concentric circles echo out to the edges of the pond. This energy radiates from you until the last ripple falls away. It is now you on the water, undisturbed and immersed in the tranquility of your setting. You drift on the surface of your unconsciousness. You feel the warmth of the water beneath you and surrounding you. The water is so soothing that you feel yourself getting heavier. You feel as though you could keep floating deeper and deeper beneath the surface until you fell asleep.

The relaxation that you feel now is beckoning you closer to rest, to deep sleep. Notice how relaxed you are in this very moment. Notice how soothing the sensations are in your body. Breathe in the relaxation that the water provides. Breathe out any tension you have.

I am going to count down from five. When I reach one, you are going to fully embrace the peace that has engulfed you and lose yourself in sleep. You will feel yourself slipping into a calm and serene rest.

Five... You think of the still surface of the pond, and how it provided safety for you, the leaf. The calm water is summoning your sleep.

Four... You feel the warmth of tranquility ripple from the top of your scalp and down your neck. It glides through your shoulders, radiates through your chest and stomach, and finally glazes over your legs. You are encompassed by this sensation.

Three... You feel your body become heavy and you softly sink in a little deeper to your consciousness. You are safe and protected.

Two... You feel yourself drift away, like your leaf on the still pond. You float away, quietly into the night.

One... You are now asleep, resting and at peace.

Breathe in, breathe out. Breathe in, breathe out. When you wake up, you will be renewed and refreshed and ready to take on the day. You will be ready to conquer the obstacles of your life now that you have conquered sleep.

Script 3

I want you to get comfortable. Listen to the sound of my voice. Let it wash over you and soothe you. Release all your stress. Release every anxiety and open your mind. Allow yourself, in body and mind, to be gently carried away. Allow yourself to be lulled into a sense of calming security. You are safe. Sway your head back and forth in the smallest of motions, just enough for you to feel the heaviness of your skull. Move it back and forth, slower and slower until you feel that you are starting to get more relaxed. When you feel the relaxation wash over you, you can slowly stop. Rest your head and feel your skull settle into the back of your head.

Take a deep breath in, hold it in your belly for one, two, three beats and then let it out. Breathe in deeply through your nose and breathe out through your mouth. Continue to breathe deeply as you slowly move your focus to your toes, warm and snuggled in your blanket. Gently curl your toes as you feel the warm sensation of peace move from the very tips of your toes upwards. The warm sensation fills your foot and slowly rolls towards your ankles and finally tingles up your calves. All the tension in your muscles floats away as the warmth moves upwards once more. It moves past your calves and swims towards the curves of your knees. It continues to travel higher and higher. Notice how your legs are feeling heavy and you are feeling calmer than before. There are no worries anymore, only this heavy warmth. Give in to the sensation that fills your body from the toes upwards. Drift into a deeper feeling of serenity and tranquility with every breath that you take.

Breathe in. Now breathe out. Slowly, gently, deeply. Breathe in. Breathe out. That peaceful warmth of relaxation continues to spread. It moves past your waist and into your stomach. It meanders over each of your ribs, wandering towards your chest. This warm feeling calms you, soothes you. All your worries begin to fade away into dust, taken away with the breeze, and you let them go, the same way you let go of your shoulders and your back as your muscles loosen even more and you feel light like air.

Ten… Your body is entirely relaxed.

Nine… You are in a peaceful, calm environment.

Eight… You can feel the warmth and love of those who care about you, enveloping your senses.

Seven… Each sound that you hear around you lulls you further into an even deeper state of relaxation.

Six… You inhale all of the good in the world with each breath you take.

Five… You exhale all the bad, blowing away all of your stress and anxiety with each breath out.

Four… You feel your body slipping even deeper.

Three… You feel your mind becoming heavier and brimming with warmth and love.

Two… Accept the peace that has engulfed you, know that it is good. Let it send you off ever deeper into the feeling of relaxation.

One… You feel yourself drifting all the way down, as deep as you can go, nearer to the bottom, towards warmth and sleep.

You are safe and you are relaxed. Allow yourself to feel safe and relaxed in this space.

Your imagination leads you to a beautiful door that shares the warmth and peace you feel. It is wooden and polished and ornately carved. It looks heavy. You place your hand on the door, your palm feels warm as you touch it. You slowly place your other palm to the door and the door easily opens. You step through the threshold.

You see you are now in dense, green woods. There is sunlight peeking through the canopy of trees high above your head. The leaves of the trees rustle in the gentle breeze. This light reminds you that you are safe. This place is where you can escape to relax. This is a soft, gentle place that you wander through. As you wander, you touch the cool, wet grass, like a sponge underfoot. In your mind's eye, you can visualize this place of tranquility and feel its serenity.

You are floating through this place, moving closer and closer to the break in the tree line. You drink in the details of your surroundings. You can see the deep green hues of the leaves and the texture of the bark, the white and yellow flowers that happily sprout up in the grass. The air smells slightly sweet. The trees stand tall above you, sentries that guard over and protect you on your journey into tranquility.

When you finally arrive, there is a clearing of trees, a lush pasture that beckons you forth. You wander to the center of the pasture and there is warmth radiating through you. You feel at home and one with the forest. You can hear sounds all around you. Leaves are rustling gently as the breeze blows against them, whispering their cadence only to you. Birds are joyously chirping somewhere in the distance, inviting you into their happiness.

Somewhere beyond this clearing is a brook, its water trickling over rocks and tinkling like bells. This place is peaceful. You can feel its tranquility dance over every nerve-ending in your body, making every ounce of your being tingle. The feeling of its loving, caressing touch on your skin makes you feel completely at peace. In this place, time has no meaning and no power. This is where you have come to center and balance your essence. Here, you have not one single worry. Here, there are no dark corners where sadness can hide, there is only truth. Your truth is warmth, peace, and light. Here, you are bathed in your truth.

As you cross the clearing and wander further along your forest path, you must take a deep breath in. You smell the freshness of the forest, its flowers and its leaves. It is breathing with you. As you exhale your tension, it exhales. You continue your walk; the grass still cools beneath your feet. You are going to notice something. It looks like a carving in the wood of one of the beautiful trees. You make your way towards it. Breathe out at the sight of it. There is a word carved neatly into the bark, just one single word.

The word is the name of this place. It is an ancient name that roots you into the core of your existence. Just the sound of the word washes you in warmth. It begins at the top of your head, trickling outwards from the center of your scalp, cascading over your ears and cheeks and down over your shoulders. It runs in rivulets over shoulders, down your arms, over your legs and through the tops of your feet. This soothing, serene word is a comfort.

Look closely at the carving in the bark and identify the word. It is a word of your choosing. This word comes to you and only you. I want you to remember this word, tuck it away in your memory, because each time you are feeling even the smallest amount of anxiety or stress that keeps you from sleep, you are going to call on this word. When you call on this word, the stress will vanish into dust, swept away on the next breeze. When you call upon this word, it will invoke this warming peace you feel. It will wash you in relaxation, and lull you into a deep, tranquil sleep.

When you call upon this word, you will remember how relaxed this forest makes you feel. How the light peeks through the canopy of leaves and how the trees stand over you and protect you. This word will call upon these guardians of your sleep and lead you into restfulness. Notice how relaxed you are in this very moment. Notice how soothing the sensations are in your body. Breathe in. Breathe out.

I am going to count down from five. When I reach one, you are going to fully embrace the peace that has engulfed you and lose yourself in sleep. You will feel yourself slipping into a calm and serene rest.

Five… You think of the word from the carving in the tree bark. Your special word. It melts away every remaining tension until your body and mind are relaxed. It is summoning your sleep.

Four… You feel the warmth of peace move from the top of your head and down your neck. It moves through your shoulders, radiates through your chest and stomach, and finally glazes over your legs.

Three… You feel your body become heavy and you softly sink in a little deeper to your consciousness. You are safe and protected.

Two… You feel yourself drift away, like a leaf on a still pond. You float away, quietly into the night.

One… You are now asleep, resting and at peace.

Breathe in, breathe out. Breathe in, breathe out. When you wake up, you will be refreshed and ready to take on the day. You will be ready to conquer the stresses of your life now that you have conquered sleep.

Chapter 14: Meditation for Deeper and Healthier Sleep

One of the best ways to really become relaxed and find the peace needed for better sleep is through the use of a visualization technique. For this, you will want to ensure that you are in a completely relaxing and comfortable place. This reading will help you be more centered on the moment, alleviate anxiety, and wind down before bed.

Listen to it as you are falling asleep, whether it's at night or if you are simply taking a nap. Ensure the lighting is right and remove all other distractions that will keep you from becoming completely relaxed.

Meditation for a Full Night's Sleep

You are laying in a completely comfortable position right now. Your body is well rested, and you are prepared to drift deeply into sleep. The deeper you sleep, the healthier you feel when you wake up.

Your eyes are closed, and the only thing that you are responsible for now is falling asleep. There isn't anything you should be worried about other than becoming well-rested. You are going to be able to do this through this guided meditation into another world.

It will be the transition between your waking life and a place where you are going to fall into a deep and heavy sleep. You are becoming more and more relaxed, ready to fall into a trance-like state where you can drift into a healthy sleep.

Start by counting down slowly. Use your breathing in fives in order to help you become more and more asleep.

Breathe in for ten, nine, eight, seven, six, and out for five, four, three, two, and one. Repeat this once more. Breathe in for ten, nine, eight, seven, six, and out for five, four, three, two, and one.

You are now more and more relaxed, more and more prepared for a night of deep and heavy sleep. You are drifting away, faster and faster, deeper and deeper, closer and closer to a heavy sleep. You see nothing as you let your mind wander.

You are not fantasizing about anything. You are not worried about what has happened today, or even farther back in your past. You are not afraid of what might be there going forward. You are not fearful of anything in the future that is causing you panic.

You are highly aware within this moment that everything will be OK. Nothing matters but your breathing and your relaxation. Everything in front of you is peaceful. You are filled with serenity and you exude calmness. You only think about what is happening in the present moment where you are becoming more and more at peace.

Your mind is blank. You see nothing but black. You are fading faster and faster, deeper and deeper, further and further. You are getting close to being completely relaxed, but right now, you are OK with sitting here peacefully.

You aren't rushing to sleep because you need to wind down before bed. You don't want to go to bed with anxious thoughts and have nightmares about the things you fear. The only thing you concern yourself with at this moment is getting nice and relaxed before it's time to start to sleep.

You see nothing in front of you other than a small white light. That light becomes a bit bigger and bigger. As it grows, you start to see that you are inside a vehicle. You are laying on your bed, everything around you are still there. Only, when you look up, you see that there is a large open window, with several computers and wheels out in front of you.

You realize that you are in a spaceship floating peacefully through the sky. It is on auto-pilot, and there is nothing that you have to worry about as you are floating up in this spaceship. You look out above you and see that the night sky is more gorgeous than you ever could have imagined.

All that surrounds you is nothing but beauty. There are bright stars twinkling against a black backdrop. You can make out some of the planets. They are all different than you would ever have imagined. Some are bright purple, others are blue. There are detailed swirls and stripes that you didn't know were there.

You relax and feel yourself floating up in this space. When you are here, everything seems so small. You still have problems back home on Earth, but they are so distant that they are almost not real. Some issues make you feel as though the world is ending, but now that the entire universe is still doing fine, no matter what might be happening in your life. You are not concerned with any issues right now.

You are soaking up all that is around you. You are so far separated from Earth, and it's crazy to think about just how much space is out there for you to explore. You are relaxed, looking around. There are shooting stars all in the distance. There are floating rocks passing by your ship. You are floating around, feeling dreamier and dreamier.

You are passing over Earth again, getting close to going back home. You are going to be sent right back into your room, falling more heavily with each breath you take back into sleep. You are getting closer and closer to drifting away.

You pass over the earth and look down to see all of the beauty that exists. The green and blue swirl together, white clouds above that make such an interesting pattern. Everything below looks like a painting. It does not look real.

You get closer and closer, floating so delicately in your small space ship. The ride is not bumpy. It is not bothering you.

You are floating over the city now. You see random lights flicker on. It doesn't look like a map anymore like when you are so high above.

You are looking down and seeing that gentle lights still flash here and there, but for the most part, the city is winding down. Everyone is drifting faster and faster to sleep. You are getting closer and closer to your home.

You see that everything is peaceful below you. The sun will rise again, and tomorrow will start. For now, the only thing you can do is prepare and rest for what might come.

You are more and more relaxed now, drifting further and further into sleep.

You are still focused on your breathing; it is becoming slower and slower. You are close to drifting away to sleep now.

When we reach one, you will drift off deep into sleep.

Chapter 15: Deep Sleep Hypnosis 2

This is going to be a thirty-minute guided hypnosis session to help you drift off into a deep and relaxing sleep. The most important thing to do while listening to this session is to keep an open mind. You must go with the flow, listen to my voice, and remember to breathe. Remember, it is not always possible to enter a light hypnotic state on the first try, but we are going to try as I guide you gently and smoothly into this state so you can fall asleep. Please bear in mind that you are not going to enter any sort of deep catatonic state. Nothing is going to be physically altered within the realm of your mind. The process of hypnosis and this guided meditation is extremely safe, and you are in control of it.

Now, I want you to get comfortable. Because you are trying to achieve deep sleep, you should be lying down, your head resting on your most comfortable pillow, and warmed by your softest blanket. Lie back and let your shoulders go slack, relaxing against the cushion of your bed. Gently close your eyes and release all the tension from your muscles. Release the tension in your arms, then your legs. Let go of the tension in your chest and in your back. All of the muscles in your body begin to feel looser and looser and your body is feeling light.

Recognize that this is a time for only you. You have set aside all of your day's activities and are ready to embrace a beautiful and peaceful sleep fully. Breathe in this moment of relaxation, where nothing else matters. There is only you in the warmth of your bed.

As you lay, I will ask you something very simple. In your mind's eye, imagination a kind of ruler or some sort of measuring device. Imagine something which can measure the depth of your own relaxation. Imagine this ruler in the front of your mind. Perhaps it is your favorite color, smooth with small painted tick marks and numbers.

Take a moment to notice where you are on your current level of relaxation. Out of a scale of 100 down to 0 being your most relaxed state. Understand that there is no right or wrong measurement to begin with. Explore your state, be honest with yourself as you measure your relaxation. What tensions do you still have left in your body? What anxieties, sadness, or pain still lingers? Very soon you are going to increase your relaxation and melt away this negativity and drift off into a peaceful sleep.

Perhaps are currently at a 60 on your scale of relaxation. Even though you may actually be lower down than that, imagine yourself moving the marker in front of you. With each deep breath, you slide the marker further down along this ruler closer and closer towards zero, towards immense relaxation. As you breathe and the marker slides down, you feel your muscles release in your arms then your legs, your back relaxes, and your chest opens like a flower, welcoming in big and tranquil breaths.

You may be aware that your sense of relaxation has expanded inside of you. Perhaps all the way down to 40 or 30. You see the marker slowly glide downwards along the scale. You feel that a wave of warmth has washed over you and you are beginning to feel your whole body becoming engulfed in the warmth of peace. As you feel your body releasing its tension even more now, you feel calmer. You have now reached a ten on your scale and gently, you take a deep breath through your nose. Let it fill your stomach until it is like to burst. Then release it.

You reach nine…You enter a peaceful, calm environment.

You reach eight…You can feel the warmth of the sun on your face. It is a reminder that you are loved.

You reach seven…Each sound that you hear, you do not deny. Instead it lulls you further and deeper into a deep state of relaxation.

You reach six…You inhale through your nose and fill your belly. You inhale all of the good things the world has to offer.

You reach five…Gently, through your nose, you release your breath. You expel any negative feelings that remain.

You reach four…You feel your body becoming lighter. Your arms and legs feel weightless and free.

You reach three… You feel your chest brimming with warmth and light.

You reach two… You accept the peace that has enveloped you. This peace welcomes you into a deepening serenity as your mind quiets.

You reach one… You feel yourself drawn towards the warmth of peaceful sleep, so close you can almost graze it with your fingertips.

You reach zero… You feel a comfort deep within you that starts in your chest and radiates outwards like a blooming flower. This comfort fills you with security and you remember that you are safe. You have released your worries and concerns, and in its place, there is warmth, light, and comfort.

Gently you are lulled by this wave of serenity. You feel yourself beginning to drift beyond zero, into a realm of warm colors. Billows of reds and pinks, yellows and oranges undulate around you in soft embraces until you float down onto a plush, cool surface.

With only your fingertips, you detect that you have landed on a grassy field. Around you, you can smell the sweet fragrance of wildflowers that have populated this clearing. Your body and mind have quieted to listen to the soft rustle of the breeze through grass and flower petals, and you remember the beauty of the earth. You breathe in through your nose a deep breath that fills your stomach. Through your nose, you slowly release it.

You recognize the warm colors from before, now painted in the sky. The reds fade into pinks seamlessly as though crafted by a painter's brush. The hues swirl into the setting sun and exude a warmth that you feel throughout your body. You are existing in this space with only beauty. You are existing without concern for time or worry. There is only you in this space and all of the tranquility it shares with you.

The pinks give way to magentas, then onto violets and dark blues. The sun sets and reveals an endless sky, sprinkled with thousands of twinkling stars. You see dustings of silver and purple in the sky. The bright sliver of moon casts its beam upon you, cascading you in comfort.

Your muscles seem to melt, going slack and welcoming sleep. The stars above you dance, twirling through the vast stretch of sky, but you are still. You allow this positive energy to enter your mind. It swells within you until you feel peace exuding from every pore. You have reached a depth of serenity that exists on the brink of sleep. Allow yourself to accept rest.

Underneath the moon, you accept rest. Soon, you begin to notice a new pleasing sensation that arrives at your arms and spreads to your legs and your back, your neck, and forehead. You recognize this sensation as a sublime floating energy entering your body. You feel a delicate tingle throughout your body, ushering in lightness and calmness. This sensation is like a soft white linen, cleansing you from the inside out. It is a warm touch of healing energy, of love and passion.

These soft vibrations rid you of tension. Anxieties are expelled. Sadness and fear no longer exist here. All of the leftover stress is now dissolving entirely, turning into dust carried off by the wind. It is melting away under the power of this healing energy. In its place there is safety and the knowledge that you are loved by whom you love. It is merely you, the stars, and the moon.

The lightness you feel swells, as if tiny balloons are attached to different parts of your body. You feel your body beginning to rise and drift upwards in the direction of the stars. Peacefulness and serenity are lifting you higher into the air into the welcoming embrace of the expansive night sky. For a brief moment you understand that you exist in the space between the earth and the sky, a realm that belongs to you and is safe from anxiety. You claim this realm as yours in which to dream. This is your dreamscape, where you float towards rest and sleep. Your realm is one of peace that connects the heavens with the ground. It is yours alone to govern, to allow only positive energy and love. You roam over the tops of trees, drift across the width of lakes, and coast above others, sleeping in their warm beds.

Your entire body now is floating higher and higher in this realm as you feel such elation inside as you realize you are now gliding through all of space. You are drifting and roaming here, no longer bound by gravity. You are now soaring like a hot air balloon, ascending higher and moving towards infinity of this welcoming expands. As you float you are letting go of everything that you no longer need. You toss away unwanted negativity. You hold on to the comfort that peace grants you.

As you become just like the pure brilliance of the stars, a beautiful shining light, you feel your spirit break free, and finally, you can float out through the entire universe. You reach out further and further into the purest wisdom, and the most loving embraces of all of the celestial beings that surround you. They are calling you to rest, to dream, to sleep, to heal. You feel yourself realigning from within..

You feel yourself moving with tranquility and mindfulness, further and further. As you wade through the stars, you feel yourself gently feeling heavier. You understand that you are drifting towards rest.

You drift through the cosmos, feeling gravity's kind tug towards the ground. Gently you float towards the earth like a leaf falls from a tree, eager to meet its rest on the ground below. You feel completely relaxed and slipping away into a restful sleep. Before you escape into your dreams, you return to your bed where you are warm and protected. Your body softly nestles under the blankets and your head snuggles into the pillow. You notice your arms and legs still feel weightless and there is a residual warm vibration throughout, a pulsing that beseeches sleep. You happily oblige.

I am going to count down from five. When I reach one, you are going to fully embrace the peace that has engulfed you and lose yourself in sleep. You will feel yourself slipping into a calm and serene rest.

Five... You think of the night sky and its expansiveness. It melts away every remaining tension until your body and mind are relaxed. It is summoning your sleep.

Four… You feel the warmth of peace move from the top of your head and down your neck. It moves through your shoulders, radiates through your chest and stomach, and finally glazes over your legs.

Three… You feel your body become heavy and you softly sink in a little deeper to your consciousness. You are safe and protected.

Two… You feel yourself drift away, like a leaf on a still pond. You float away, quietly into the night.

One… You are now asleep, resting and at peace.

Breathe in, breathe out. Breathe in, breathe out. When you wake, you will be refreshed and ready to take on the day. You will be ready to conquer the stresses of your life now that you have conquered sleep.

Chapter 16: Overcome Mental blocks to Lose Weight

Metabolism

Metabolism is the constant process that your body uses to keep everything functioning. Your metabolism is always running, even when you're sleeping.

Some people have a faster metabolism than others, which is the result of genetics and someone's lifestyle. Although there's nothing you can do about your genetics, there are ways to impact your lifestyle and give your metabolism a boost to keep it up in high gear.

How can you improve your metabolism?

Since the metabolism's base rate is set by genetics, there's no quick way to alter it; it cannot be modified without making some long-term lifestyle changes.

If you're looking to speed up your metabolism, then there are a few habits you can add, improve, or modify throughout the day. Working out, hydrating, and eating right can help with your overall health, but there are also other specific changes you can foster to give it a boost.

Apart from getting in more muscle-building or endurance workouts and eating better during the day, another critical habit to run your metabolism properly is not ignoring the most important meal of the day: breakfast.

People tend to underrate how important breakfast is, we go all night without food, and our body can approach a fasting state, an episode where our body will withhold calories if we wait too long to eat after waking up.

What can slow your metabolism?

If it's possible to speed up your metabolism, then it's also possible -- and far easier -- to slow it down. Many habits are easy to fall into, which can make your metabolism run at a slower pace. One of these happens in the late hours of the night and involves what you're not doing: getting enough quality sleep.

Sleep deprivation is one of the biggest, and yet overlooked epidemics in society. It is one of the most significant factors that people seem to forget about. Even if someone eats well and exercises, if they don't get adequate sleep (in particular deep sleep which involves the REM phase), then their metabolism won't run properly.

Stress can also indirectly lead to severe problems that affect your metabolism. People with high amounts of cortisol, a stress hormone, tend to be overweight, and being overweight slows down metabolism.

Lowering your cortisol levels can start a chain reaction that can push your metabolism to run more efficiently.

What Does Your Metabolism do Over Time?

Believe it or not, metabolism goes through the aging process as well. As your metabolism slows, your continuous eating habits and exercise choices become more critical.

While the cause for this is not clear yet, women entering menopause will experience a slower metabolism. They can find it challenging to stay at a healthy weight, which makes diet, exercise, and rest vital to healthy aging.

How the Mind Controls the Metabolism?

We build our beliefs over a lifetime. Beliefs create ideas and ideas produce thoughts; these thoughts, in turn, generate emotions, and these emotions, finally, impact organ function. At every moment of your life, you create your health through beliefs. The mind chooses what it wants to connect to, based on ideas that it's formed. Your mind is the most potent tool you have for creating a healthy metabolism function. Is the mind the main engine that drives metabolism function.

The choices we make in terms of beliefs support the highest level of metabolism function. Remember this simple truth: "If you always associate with the good, you will become the good. If you associate with the negative, you become the negative." Sometimes, it isn't effortless to give up a belief. But if we replace the negative ones that impact health, we can make tremendous healing progress. You can boost your metabolism function daily by choosing positive, kind, healthful beliefs. And when beliefs change, the same eyes can look at the same reality differently, therefore see different things. Then, different outcomes are possible.

How to Overcome Mental Blocks

We are prisoners of our minds. Our mind, in turn, is responsible for the normal and healthy functioning of the body. Grounding our thought patterns with pessimism only return feelings of negativity, which eventually affect one's mental health. This is because the latter issue only contributes to mood and anxiety symptoms.

Yet, what is this phenomenon called "meditation"? Meditation is a practice that involves the application of various techniques such as breathing and mindfulness to achieve a calm mental state and train focus and attention. The primary purpose of the practice is to help you observe your feelings and emotions without judgment with the benefit that you will get to understand them well. Therefore, meditation does not make you a holy person or a different person, but it has the potential to if you wish to take the path.

What is not meditation? Meditation is not a practice meant to make you high or zone out or even have bizarre experiences. Many people carry this notion around with them. It would be a good idea to dispel some of these thoughts before getting yourself to start the practice lest you feel deceived. Meditation is an avenue to train your mind in awareness.

Why Practice Meditation and Affirmations?

Some personal development coaches see positive affirmations as the backbone of personal development. While the constant repetition of affirmations to yourself causes your subconscious mind to absorb and act on it, the effect can almost double when combined with meditation.

Meditation is effective in communicating with you and charging your batteries. It relieves you of stress, finds your center, and has many health benefits. You have no reason not to meditate. However, many people find it difficult to enter the mental state required for meditation. Although the basic meditation techniques are quite simple, they are required to calm the mind, which is something that your mind is not used to. With our chaotic modern life, our minds have mastered the art of simultaneously juggling thoughts, and we find it more challenging to let go when we need to.

Repeating affirmations is a great way to calm and transform that turbulent state of mind into a more peaceful way of meditating. These statements will stimulate your mind to prepare for meditation and take it to the next level by helping you to:

- Focus on the present. You will observe that you are less likely to think about future or past events when you focus on the breath and the present moment. Over time, this will allow you to enter deeper and take your meditation to a whole new level.

- Calm your thoughts and release stress tension. You will have more control over your thoughts; and able to detach from stressful events. During meditations, your mind will be more relaxed, and your body will be deeply relaxed, allowing you to be more focused on your meditation.

This is one that quickly enters a deeper meditative state. With time, you find it easier to clear your mind and enter into a deep meditative state as soon as you take a position.

Meditation + positive affirmations = success

Words, positive or not, have no value in themselves. Every word we say, hear or think evokes an image, a sound, a taste, or a feeling that belongs to us. Every morning, when you wake up with a thousand thoughts in your head and repeat "Today I will make the best day of my life" it will bring you, and you will feel more energetic and positive, but how long will it take? Hardly an hour!

No, there is nothing wrong with a positive choice. The problem lies in the mood. Your subconscious and the conscious mind is so full of continuous "conversations" of random thoughts that you do not allow the positive affirmation to evoke a deep connection between your mind and soul.

In this case, the positive affirmation becomes the menu: you know what it can offer and also the flavor. To taste the food, you must provide an empty plate in the form of a calm and receptive mind.

.

How do you use positive affirmations in meditation?

Make sure your mind is entirely calm and deeply relaxed. You can listen to relaxing music for meditation if you have a hard time keeping your mind calm; you can try to focus on a particular object nearby.

Once you feel relaxed and in tune with your feelings, begin repeating your choice of positive affirmation. Remember that it is best to choose a statement with which you can relate deeply. For example, instead of saying, "I will lose weight," choose, "I will lose 10 kilos in 3 months." It will help your mind focus on what needs to be done when it needs to be done, and whatever it is you have to do, you have the power to do it.

Meditation unleashes the power of positive thinking, which in turn points the laser at your positive affirmations. A positive attitude is nothing more than a manifestation of positive thinking, and to think positively, you must first believe in positivity.

Another technique is to record your positive affirmation and then meditate. Use lots of energy and positivity when recording your statements; say it as you really want and believe it. Visualization is a potent tool too. If you have photos that you can link to your affirmation choice, please keep them for yourself. Otherwise, use the power of your imagination and create a corresponding image.

A common problem faced by even the most seasoned meditation practitioners with positive affirmations is the doubt and negativity they often hint at. For someone who has eaten comfortably for years and has not followed any diet, it would be hard to believe that you will lose 10 pounds in 3 months. Slowly, this bubble of uncertainty and negativity begins to expand; This is where you should avoid and restore all negative thoughts.

While the chances of random negative thoughts popping up will significantly decrease if you meditate before reciting affirmations, it doesn't go away entirely. You will make a conscious effort to reject it and repeat the statement with additional conviction and energy.

Affirmations and meditation seem to go hand in hand. For essential respiratory meditations, it is best to make short statements. In this way, they are easy to remember, and you will not be out of breath if you repeat them. Be sure to keep your words positive and in the present. Tell yourself silent confirmation with each breath. And at each expiration, feel the increasing serenity that the statement you have chosen brings. Simple and effective meditations can be created by confirming liberation and acceptance.

Chapter 17: Guided Meditations

Meditation for Healthier Habits

Visualization, suggestion combined with meditation, is an easy way to make positive and powerful personal changes. If you combine meditation with positive affirmation, you will begin to change the way you feel, think, and act. This relaxation exercise will help you change and improve the way you feel. However, the time taken to see the effects differs from person to person. Let's begin…

Sit or lie down comfortably.

Stretch your back and then put your shoulders backward to open the rib cage.

Feel your shoulder muscles relax.

Close your eyes.

Relax your body and empty your mind.

Take ten slow but deep breaths.

Concentrate on the breath.

Feel it getting slower and deeper

Feel relaxed as every tension goes away.

Relax your neck and shoulders again.

<Pause a minute for reflection>

Imagine being happy, being successful, winning, being loved, laughing, feeling good.

Relax your forehead, mouth and eyes.

Let a soft smile appear on your face as you feel a calm enter your mind.

<Pause a minute for reflection>

<MEDITATION CLOSING>

Then say the following words:

- I'm a good person
- I do what is right.
- I have integrity
- Whatever life presents is a useful experience that will only make me wiser, stronger, and more tolerant.
- I eat and drink good things.

- I am what I eat and drink
- I focus on the joy in my life
- I am what I see, touch and hear positive things.
- I am compassionate, loving and caring.
- I am strong enough to understand that the behavior of others is about them, not me.
- I help others when I can
- I exercise because I enjoy it.
- I smile and laugh because I am happy.
- I help other people. After all, they are all good people, like me.
- I'm what I say I am
- I am

Meditative affirmations are a centuries-old way of gaining control over our feelings and behaviors.

Meditation for Positive Thinking

This hypnotherapy experience will allow you to easily fall asleep while your calm and relaxed mind can enjoy listening along to a series of beneficial suggestions, all of which are in the form of positive affirmations to enhance your health, wealth, and happiness.

You will find that there is nothing overly complicated in this session. Allow yourself to drift into hypnosis and then away into your dreams.

During this restful time ahead, your conscious mind will inevitably wander but your subconscious mind will continue to listen to my voice.

As you settle in and lay your head on the pillow, you can be reassured that all of these suggestions will speak powerfully to your subconscious mind. It makes no difference whether you remember or forget the pleasant suggestions in this session. You can trust in my voice to permeate your subconscious being while you fall into the deep state of hypnosis.

As you are preparing to relax, take a moment to reassure yourself that all hypnosis is self-hypnosis, which means that you remain in control throughout the entirety of this session. If something from the outside world requires your presence at any time, you can simply open your eyes, and the hypnosis will be over.

But for now, you can continue to relax, and allow the noise and distractions of the outside world to continue to fade away…gently into the night.

Because this time is the perfect time to let go and let it all drift away…

This is the perfect time to relax…

If they aren't already, close your eyes lightly.

Throughout this time, there is no need to do anything. There is no need to worry about things that happened today or things that might happen tomorrow. Right now, all you need to do is to be here, in your body, on your bed, letting your mind do what it needs to do to relax for a good night's sleep.

Thank yourself for taking this time for self-care. You deserve a night of restful sleep and to wake up feeling refreshed and ready for the day. This is one thing that you can do that is just for yourself. No guilt, no worries.

Know that whatever worries you and stops you from sleeping won't be fixed by keeping you awake.

Know that no matter how you slept last night, or the night before, you can sleep well tonight. This is the only night that matters.

Just let yourself go…

Lie still as you allow the stress to fade away.

<Pause a minute for reflection>

Each time you find your mind drifting, notice where it's gone and gently tell yourself to come back to being right here, right now. There is no need to judge what your mind is thinking about, or that you have become distracted. This is what our brains are designed to do.

Now, take a deep breath.

And exhale.

Take a deep breath.

And exhale.

Take a deep breath and feel the air as it flows through your nostrils, down into your lungs and fully into your abdomen. Breathe in as deeply as you can.

<Pause a minute for reflection>

As your body relaxes, it may begin to feel heavy. Feel how it rests on the bed. You are supported in this meditation by the things around you. They hold you and allow your mind to do the work needed to unclutter your mind.

Like your breath, your body may hold areas of tension that distract you. When you notice tension, try to relax those muscles. You may find that a small stretch and release of the muscles helps reduce the tension. This doesn't have to be a big movement. Just enough to allow your muscles to fall back down into a restful state.

This is something that resets the muscle memory into one of relaxation rather than tension.

Now, take a deep breath.

And exhale.

Deep breath.

And exhale.

<Pause a minute for reflection>

Now, I will count down from 10 to 1.

With each passing number, you will feel yourself falling deeper and deeper into a peaceful state of relaxation.

With each passing number, you will feel your body grow increasingly heavier. Allow this feeling to wash over you, and allow the tension from your muscles to fade away. Allow yourself to relax.

10.

9.

8.

7.

6.

5.

4.

3.

2.

1.

I am learning to relax to the deepest I can go.

I am learning to relax to the deepest I can go.

With each breath, I fall deeper into a state of relaxation.

With each breath, I fall deeper into a state of relaxation.

I slowly release all control.

I slowly release all control.

<Pause a minute for reflection>

<MEDITATION CLOSING>

- I am the architect of my life.
- I am unique.
- I am happy.
- I am successful.
- I am positive.
- I am special.
- I am in full control, relaxed, and comfortable.
- I am now in the perfect place, and this is the perfect time to rest and sleep.
- I welcome dreams of positivity and abundance.

- I welcome relaxation with a heart full of gratitude.
- With each breath, I dive deeper into a state of relaxation.
- With each breath, I dive deeper into a state of relaxation.
- Positive energy comes to me easily and effortlessly.
- Positive energy comes to me easily and effortlessly.
- The more I let go, the deeper I relax.
- The more I let go, the deeper I relax.

Meditation to Cope During Difficult Times

Sit comfortably with your legs crossed and your arms placed on your thigh's palms facing up

(5 seconds)

Take three deep breaths and exhale completely with each breath.

(30 seconds)

Keep breathing deeply allowing your body to become relaxed.

(60 seconds)

Now, bring your attention to the challenges you are facing. Without thinking too much about them, just identify them one by one.

(20 seconds)

How are you feeling? Are you mad, sad, stressed, in pain, or sorrowful? Identify the emotions that stand out for you in this moment.

(10 seconds)

Realize that these emotions are a manifestation of the chemical process taking place in your body. Therefore, notice them without judgement or getting involved in them.

(15 seconds)

Do not try to push them away either. Instead become a curious observer. Notice how intense they are. Are they manifesting on a specific part of the body? For instance, can your feel a heaviness at your solar plexus, or do your shoulders feel tight? Or is your heart feeling a bit faster. Have you lost your smile and your jaw is tightly clenched and lips tightly closed? Become aware of the parts of the body that these emotions are manifesting.

(30 seconds)

Whatever feelings you are experiencing, you do not need to be ashamed of them just because you perceive them as negative feelings. Be open to them. See them as a way of your body responding to various circumstances and happenings. It is alright, you are human, and you are allowed to feel how you are felling in this moment.

(60 seconds)

Now, begin to deepen your breaths.

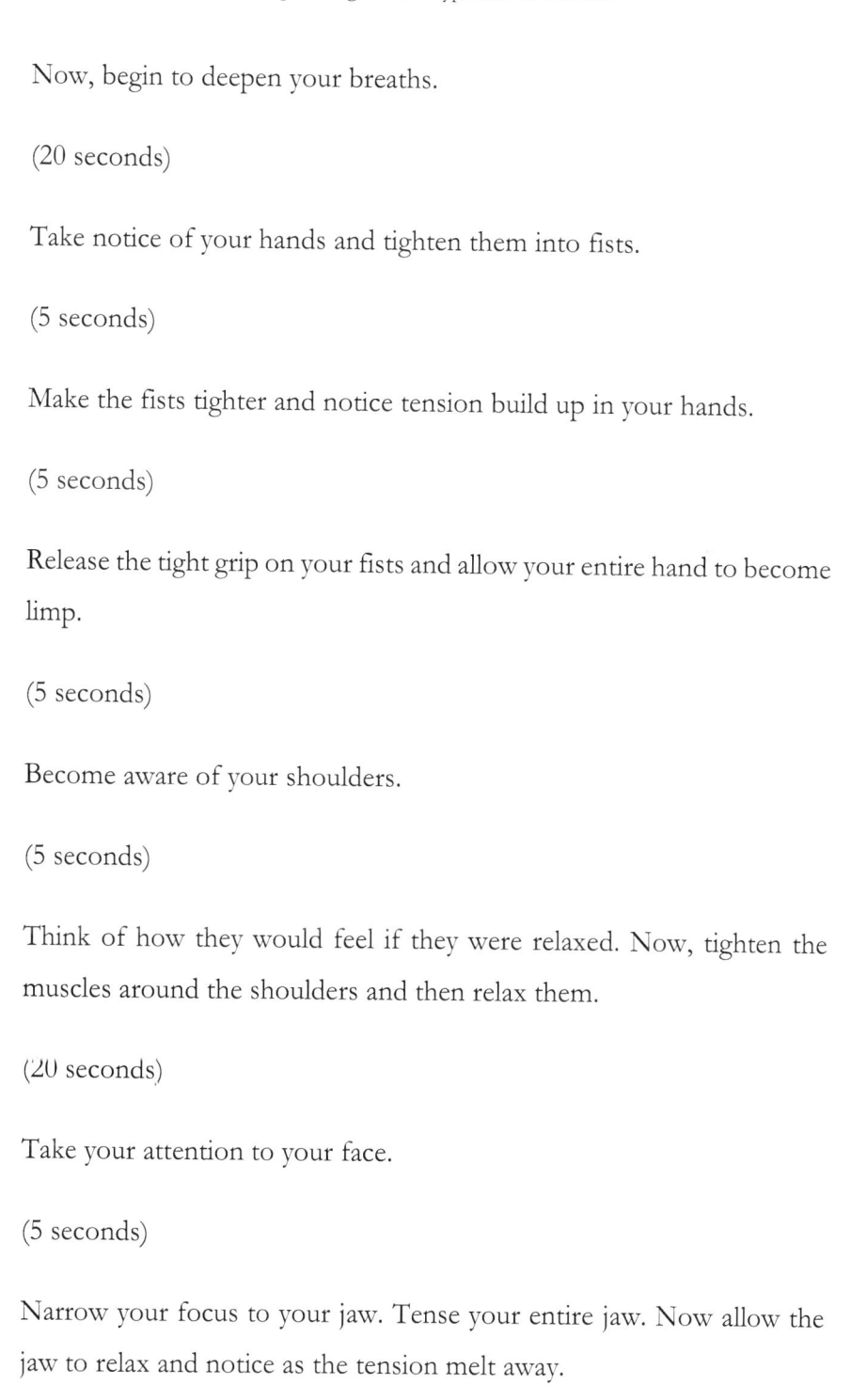

(20 seconds)

Take notice of your hands and tighten them into fists.

(5 seconds)

Make the fists tighter and notice tension build up in your hands.

(5 seconds)

Release the tight grip on your fists and allow your entire hand to become limp.

(5 seconds)

Become aware of your shoulders.

(5 seconds)

Think of how they would feel if they were relaxed. Now, tighten the muscles around the shoulders and then relax them.

(20 seconds)

Take your attention to your face.

(5 seconds)

Narrow your focus to your jaw. Tense your entire jaw. Now allow the jaw to relax and notice as the tension melt away.

(5 seconds)

Now scan your whole body and search for hidden stress in the muscles. Relax every area that you can senses tension.

(120 seconds)

Scan one more time to see if there is any part of the body that is still tensed even if just a little bit. Tighten the body part and allow it to relax.

(60 seconds)

Now scan the whole body from your head to your toes. Take a deep breath in and tightly squeeze all the parts of your body. Hold your breath in and continue to squeeze your muscles some more. Begin to exhale slowly as you relax the entire body.

Become aware of how your body is feeling now.

You are gaining control of your negative emotions.

You are no longer hiding these emotions.

You have taken a step to allow yourself to feel them but not giving them control over your life.

Remember that allowing yourself to acknowledge these negative feelings is an act of courage.

(10 seconds)

Once again, begin to take deep breaths.

(20 seconds)

With the expansion of every inhale, allow your body to create room in your heart for positive emotions. With the contraction of every exhale become aware of your ability to cope with difficult times and emotions.

(5 seconds)

Keep breathing in and out as you allow your body to create more space for grace, strength and courage.

(60 seconds)

Now, allow your breathing to adapt to its normal rhythm and just observe it.

(60 seconds)

Think of a time, you were delighted and at peace. When was it? How was life then. How did you feel? Remember that moment in details.

(20 seconds)

Allow yourself to relive that moment and for the emotions you felt then to fill your body and mind.

(20 seconds)

Let the memory and emotions of that time remind you that no matter all the negative emotions of fear, distress, doubt, hatred, overwhelm, and mistrust you are feeling right now, you will overcome and experience joy and peace again.

(10 seconds)

Think of a person, place, or experience related that brings you joy. Visualize it or the person in details and let the joy of thinking about it or them fill your heart.

(20 seconds)

Think about what is most important in your life. Maybe it is your family, career, friends, or relationship?

Despite these difficult times, you still have something to be grateful for. Identify what is going well in these areas of your life and express gratitude for it. Let it encourage you that all is not lost, that you will overcome.

(60 seconds)

Take a deep breath and hold it in. Allow your heart and mind to fill with gratitude. Exhale gently as you continue to express gratitude for even the smallest things that you take for granted like your heart beating or your ability to talk among others.

While things are difficult at this moment, you can still choose to make the most out of life. Be deliberate about thinking empowering thoughts that sooth you, support you and encourage you. Choose to be compassionate and kind to yourself. And manage your time and energy in a way that allow you to cope the best way possible.

(20 seconds)

Visualize yourself getting to the other side of whatever difficulty you are experiencing. How does it feel to have surmounted this challenge or obstacle? You will be stronger and wiser on the other end. And for that reason, you choose not to give up on yourself or to allow yourself get drained by all the negative emotions you are feeling.

(20 seconds)

Make a promise to yourself to be kind to yourself and be grateful even though for just one thing amid the challenge you are facing.

(10 seconds)

As we wind up this meditation, repeat the following affirmations:

1. I feel the fear, the doubt and the difficulty but I choose to show up everyday
2. I have what it takes to overcome these challenges
3. Even though I am faced with a difficult situation, I completely love and accept myself

4. I offer myself compassion, love and kindness during these tough times

5. I allow myself to feel the pain but not allow it to maim my spirit and my being.

6. This too shall pass

7. Better days are coming

8. I choose to hang in there with optimism

Understand that difficult moments will pass. They may seem like they are fixed in your life at the moment, but with time, they shall pass. Nothing is permanent and this too shall pass. So, hang in there. Muster the courage and strength you need. You will overcome.

(20 seconds)

Chapter 18:
Love Your Body, Love Your Soul

Taking care of your body is taking care of your soul! You show yourself the highest love for yourself when you take care of your body. We all want love! The great paradox is that to receive love, you must first choose to accept it. To accept the love of others, you must learn as before: you must first love yourself to learn how to receive love and pass it on to others. Loving yourself really makes you kinder to others!

However, loving ourselves is extremely difficult to do. In my experience, I see this problem over and over again! It is the most common problem among many people! Without love for yourself, you will always wait for love to come. You may wonder, why am I so unlovable? It's because you don't love yourself enough!

When I talk about loving yourself, when I broach the subject of loving your body, I can already feel the pain. Since you prefer to ignore the fact that you are a physical being, your lack of self-love pours into your body. Loving your body is very, very difficult in our culture, with perfection as the highest goal. So instead, you can choose to ignore your body, as if it wasn't part of you. Let your mind take over, ignoring whatever your poor body is trying to tell you.

To have comprehensive and integral health, you MUST learn to love your body and therefore to listen to it! You need to access your body and its wisdom through the sensing mechanisms of the right brain rather than the thinking of the left brain, rationalizing the mechanisms. You must access your intuition!

When you love your body, you are displaying at the highest act of self-love. Taking care of your body, you take care of your whole being; you take care of your body-mind-soul. If the goal is full body-mind-soul integration, how can you integrate if you disconnect from your body and treat it as a separate being?

You disconnect from your body every day when you get up too late, feed on sugar and processed foods, can't exercise, and work too long. When you do that, you ignore it as part of yourself.

I call the body "intentionally" because we often see our bodies as if they were a separate and distinct entity from us. If you treat your body with love, you are healing the soul through the body. It is truly a spiritual process, as the body-mind-soul is one, whether you choose to acknowledge it or not.

Every little act you do to take care of your body also means taking care of your mind and soul. Any small step you take to start the change will earn you thousands of rewards. As a result of taking care of your body, your mental health will improve, and you will feel better overall. It will create space in your life for you, and it will create a balance in your life in all things: your financial affairs, your work life, and your home life.

This will create positive energy and spread to everyone around you!

Is your Weight your Barometer for Happiness?

I understood that my weight could sometimes be a direct barometer of my happiness. It tells me that every time I start gaining weight, I am too stressed for anything. My self-love is gone, and I'm disconnected from myself, disconnected from happiness, and disconnected from love. I immediately focus on my methods to lose weight healthily before my weight gets out of control.

The stress hormone you secrete, cortisol that prepares you for emergencies, also helps you retain fat in an emergency. Have you ever wondered why when you're happy, you can eat a mountain of food and not gain weight, but when you're stressed, even just looking at that dessert makes you gain weight? It is from the stress hormone cortisol. It is because the need to fill the void when you are emotionally distressed is so high that the body pumps cortisol, trying to prepare for the emergency.

Being always stressed and emotionally distressed leads you to continually try to satisfy the emotional need, to fill the void in your life. You eat carbohydrates to feel better because carbohydrates help the body to release the wellness hormone called serotonin.

A vicious circle follows. Some call it the stress cycle. Stress leads to cortisol secretion and causes carbohydrate binge eating to make you feel better. Therefore, more food causes more distress and increases cortisol secretion and fat storage. Which leads to eating even more...

The connection between food and love is great. It was the way we all came into the world, finding a mother, and her love as a source of food, a source of love and warmth. Without the love, warmth, and touch of a human being, despite being fed, a child will suffer. Love and food education go hand in hand.

The association between love and food is so strong that you think you will feed when you taste your favorite ice cream. You think you pay attention to yourself because you deserve it and you are giving yourself love, but the temporary feeling of immediate gratification soon turns to remorse and hatred for the lack of willpower, sometimes immediately after consumption.

An indication of genuine care for yourself is if you still feel good about what you did the next day. I don't remember feeling good about the giant bowl of ice cream I had the night before, but I do feel good after exercise or after meditation.

I never said after exercising: "God, I wish I hadn't walked three miles!". And after a lovely meditation, I always feel fresh and rejuvenated. After each activity that brings you joy and satisfaction, you feel that you have taken care of yourself, which makes you feel rested and renewed. This is true love for yourself.

I never regret a meditation or hypnosis session. It is good for my soul, helping me to connect with myself to recharge and rejuvenate. The benefits of hypnosis and meditation are phenomenal self-love activities.

If you don't take care of your body, you are ignoring its importance to your mental, emotional, and spiritual health. You are saying that you don't love yourself enough to take care of your body-mind-soul. Show your amount of love for yourself to the world through the way you treat yourself.

Positive Affirmations for Weight Loss

The journey to weight loss is both physical and mental. If not more. This explains why we must prepare our minds for effective weight loss. And better yet, prepare for a successful life on it. Affirmation is one way for us to develop our mind for effective weight loss.

Affirmation is simply a statement you say. We affirm what we want in life with our thoughts and beliefs. The universe works in a way that it brings us experiences that resonate with our thoughts. For instance, if you think that losing weight is too difficult, it will be. If you think it is exhilarating but achievable, it will be. Your thoughts either help you succeed or stop you.

Using affirmations is an effort to deliberately taking charge of your thoughts. Affirmation works to neutralize unconscious beliefs that block your progress and create a conducive environment for weight loss success. However, affirmations alone may not be enough to remove deep-seated beliefs. These can best be resolved through self-hypnosis. Here are some of the best weight-loss affirmations that will help you lose weight:

My goal to lose weight is to feel healthier, happier and look better in my clothes.

- I recognize that there are other things in life that give me long-term happiness and that binging is not one of them.

- I intend to control myself, build my discipline, and not give up when I want to.

- I am committed to living a healthier life.

- I eat healthily and lose weight quickly.

- I deserve to be thin. I am worthy of being healthy and eating healthy food.

- I love and accept myself. I like my company. They are much more than my body.

- I love eating good food, exercising, resting and being in the company of great people.

- I am beautiful and eating too much prevents me from seeing it.
- I let myself be slim and healthy. With ease, I reach my perfect figure.
- I am worthy of loving myself.
- I am on my way to happiness and overeating is just another obstacle to overcome.
- I am satisfied with my physical appearance.
- I am human and uncontrolled cravings are normal, but I have to submit to them.
- I have overcome these cravings before and can do it again.
- I choose the perfect health for me. I eat it healthy and lose weight easily.
- I deserve more than short-term satisfaction; I deserve long-term happiness.
- Every day I get a step closer to my ideal weight. So, I feel bright, healthy, satisfied and happy.
- If I overcome these cravings, I will be one step closer to my goal and each step counts.

- This moment is my new opportunity. I choose perfect thoughts, perfect health and perfect life for me.

Say your affirmations with joy and enthusiasm. Stand in front of the mirror and say it out loud. Have fun while doing it! Feel the joy flow through your body as you say your affirmations.

Affirmations for Self-Love

Affirmations are statements that we use to induce a positive mood. With affirmations of self-love, we reaffirm our belief that we every right to love ourselves. Life is full of relationships. Relations with our siblings, parents, friends, and lovers. While there are many different relationships on the journey of life, there is only one person who will be there with you for life, and that's you.

Of all the different affirmations that exist, the affirmation of self-love re among the most important. There is nothing better than loving yourself. After all, only you have been there with yourself. From the day you were born until the day of your death.

This is why self-love affirmations are so meaningful. They motivate us to be happy with who we are and to love ourselves. We can do what we want as long as we believe in ourselves. You won't get anywhere without a little love for yourself because you don't feel like you deserve it.

Remember that the key is not just saying the words, but also believing in every word you say. Because even if the only person who loves and appreciates you is yourself, it is more than enough. Here are some of the best affirmations for self-love:

- I respect myself
- I am pretty
- I am happy
- I am fantastic
- I am free from worries and regrets
- I feel great about who I am
- I am special
- I am adorable
- I forgive myself and I accept myself
- I am a nice person
- I am calm and peaceful
- I love myself, unconditionally.
- I love looking at my reflection
- I deserve to live in peace and love myself
- I let go of negative feelings and thoughts about myself and accept all that is good.

- I love myself from head to toe in and out
- I only have good feelings about myself
- I like my company
- I am changing for the better
- I choose only positive thoughts and feelings about myself.

Affirmations for Self-Esteem

The term self-esteem describes a person's general sense of self-worth. In simple terms, it's how much you value and appreciate yourself.

Having low self-esteem can make people lack confidence, depressed, make bad decisions, or even getting into toxic relationships. Sometimes, the individual may also exhibit a personality disorder in which he has too much self-esteem.

Why is self-esteem important?

Self-esteem would play an essential role by motivating us to achieve success throughout our life. This means having low self-esteem can prevent you from reaching your full potential. Low self-esteem harms your performance. When you have low self-esteem, you will find it difficult to believe in your abilities and the possibility of achieving success. Likewise, having a healthy self-esteem can help you face life with more confidence in your skills and a positive attitude. Here are some of the best positive affirmations for self-esteem:

- My life is beautiful and rewarding.

- I love who I am

- I choose to be happy, regardless of my situation

- I have been blessed with the health, joy, happiness and abundance.

- I have confidence in the abilities and skills.

- I am loved and respected wherever I am

- I am creative, self-sufficient and hard-working.

- I am generously rewarded because people appreciate my abilities.

- I am a unique individual and I don't need to test myself with anyone.

- I appreciate the things that I have. I rejoice in the love I receive.

- I am not rooted in one place; I have the possibility to change.

- I deserve all the good things in life.

- I am a solution maker. I see challenges as an opportunity to grow.

- I am grateful for all the extraordinary things in my life.

- I would live my life to the fullest; I'm not a prisoner to my past mistakes.

- I am flexible and adapt to challenges and experiences.

- I am responsible for my actions and decisions.

- I always hope for the best and think positively.
- I am strong and confident.
- I am sure it would be successful. It's already written in the stars.

Simple Daily Good Habits

I believe that today's life is the sum of your daily habits over time. Your health, your mood, and even your success is a direct result of your habits. The activities you do repeatedly determine who you are at the end of the day. Everything you do regularly shapes your life. Therefore, the practices you adopt will either make or break you. By gradually developing good habits, you can eventually change your whole life.

It may be particularly helpful to analyze the behaviors you portray in your daily life carefully. You will come to see that some of these activities are very helpful and will help you get closer to your goals. However, some other behaviors are only disruptive and can only lead you astray. More often, bad habits enter your life without you even noticing. But after constant repetition, the negative behavior now becomes a bad habit that has an impact on your life.

One way to break bad habits is to replace them with better ones. By beginning to replace unfavorable behavior patterns with more favorable ones, it is possible to build a better future gradually. Even small changes can make a difference. Here are over 30 good habits that can help you transform your life.

All of these habits are easy to implement but exceptionally powerful.

Wake up early

The key to maximum performance is getting enough sleep. As such, there is a huge gap between being a night bird to an early riser. Among many other benefits, waking up early can significantly increase your productivity. By going to bed at a reasonable time and getting up early, you can easily balance your life and enjoy a higher level of concentration.

Prioritize

Rather than trying to tackle multiple tasks at once, it better to prioritize. Prioritize your goals and recreational activities at the same time. Focus first on the main activities.

Practice gratitude.

If you can be grateful for the smallest aspect of your life, you can become increasingly freed from painful experiences.

This will help you find joy in what you have and will make you less dependent on the purchase of material goods. Cultivating an attitude of gratitude is one of the best habits for a happier and fuller life.

Motivate yourself.

Motivation is what fuels your effort to achieve success in every aspect of life. If you can motivate yourself, it will feed your efforts. Remember that no one else can light this fire but you. Others may try to motivate you, but the fire soon goes out.

So, you must motivate yourself effectively.

Visualize.

To achieve success, we must visualize success and have a strong belief that it is possible. By seeing the desired results, you can train your subconscious mind to help you take the necessary steps to reach your goals. This is a simple technique that gives impressive results.

Think positively.

The way you think you can make or break you. Positive thinking works to feed your mind that you can find a solution despite the obstacles. Positive thinking helps you expect positive results, even when you have challenges. Besides, positive thinking helps to improve your overall health and reduces stress.

Learn to say no.

Your ability to say NO is very crucial if you want to have a healthy, focused, and productive life. Saying "no" has to do with your ability to avoid distractions to stay focused on your dreams and goals.

Learning to say "no" will help you spend more time on what's important in your life.

Set goals.

If you have no life goals, you are more likely to walk in different directions without reaching your destination. SMART goals are needed to direct all your actions in one direction. They will guide you and give you the concentration you need to overcome obstacles on the road to success. The high power of targets can best be exploited by looking at your goals.

Also, get in the habit of regularly checking or adjusting your goals.

Meditate.

Studies have repeatedly shown that meditation can profoundly improve many aspects of our lives. It can help relieve us of stress and reduce depression. Meditation can also help you overcome fear-based thinking.

Exercise.

It's no news that regular exercise offers a lot of benefits. Not only does it keep your body healthy, but it can also help improve your mental health.

By exercising regularly, you can increase your energy and overall mood.

Live consistently

Sometimes it can be challenging to be consistent, but you will almost always regret it later if you sacrifice your ideals for other people or your professional achievements. Instead, live with integrity and act consistently.

Eat healthily

An unbalanced and unhealthy eating habit can make dealing with everyday problems a lot more complicated. By eating healthily, you will not only provide your body with the necessary nutrients, but you are also laying the foundation for a happier and fulfilling life.

Make decisions effectively

Your success in every aspect of life depends largely on your ability to make the right decisions effectively. Try to make decisions that balance speed and reasonableness. Instead of wasting time continuously planning, act on your choices, and make changes along the way.

Create lists

Writing a list of all the responsibilities you must address can go a long way in setting priorities. The list also gives you a good overview of the activities you face.

This will help you better assess the urgency and importance of individual tasks.

Stretch regularly

Stretching is a habit that can be easily developed.

This does not only increase your flexibility, but it also helps your body cope better with day-to-day challenges, such as being in an office chair for too long.

Write

Writing down your thoughts can help you think hard about your life experiences. It is a fantastic habit that many appreciate very much because it helps them clarify their ideas.

Use affirmations

Positive affirmations can go a long way in reducing the limiting impact of negative thoughts. This encourages and increases your courage to continue pursuing your goals.

Cook more often

In times of increased workload and deadlines, it is even more difficult to find time to cook. You can make a huge difference in your life by developing the habit of cooking.

Not only is it good to know that you have prepared your food, but the whole process is also relaxing and helps you become more aware of what you are eating.

Feed your inspiration and motivation

By regularly surrounding yourself with inspiring materials, you can refill the internal fire that keeps you going.

Smile more often

When you smile more often, the muscles in your body take a position that your brain associates with positive emotions, such as joy and happiness So, get in the habit of smiling even if you don't want to.

Reconnect with nature

As children, we spent most of the day outdoors on the street or in nature. As we age, this habit is slowly but gradually replaced by other activities. It can be extremely joyful to reconnect with nature and spend more time outdoors.

Under promise

Instead of making promises you can't keep, try to keep expectations low and only make promises you can keep. It will help you avoid the pressure of meeting high expectations, as you know that this is almost impossible.

Do something new every day

Get used to interrupting your routines and making refreshing changes in your life.

Eat mindfully

By eating mindfully, you not only pay more attention to what you eat, but you will also eat less. So instead of eating as fast, try to eat more consciously. Enjoy what you eat and chew more deeply.

Eat healthy snacks

Snacks can be incredibly difficult. However, you don't have to stop snacking completely. Instead, replace unhealthy snacks like cookies, chocolate, donuts, and chips with healthier alternatives like fruits, nuts, and vegetables.

Find time for yourself

Taking out time for yourself every day can incredibly increase your happiness. The time you spend with yourself will not only allow you chase the things you are passionate about but also help your clear your mind.

Let the day end

The importance of gradually ending the day cannot be overemphasized. Instead of working or watching television before bed, rest for at least half an hour.

During this period, you can practice meditation. You will notice the impact this has on your ability to fall asleep and the quality of your sleep.

Take advantage of short breaks

We are so used to technology that we no longer take advantage of the short breaks that life offers us. Not only is this fun, but it also prevents you from making a real break. You can avoid this by getting into the habit of maximizing your short breaks. Relax and do nothing for a few minutes. You will see how refreshing a short break can be.

Explore

There is so much more to discover that you could spend your whole life exploring the world and all that it contains. But it is crucial to take the time necessary for this exploration of consciousness. Even if you are an intentional, disciplined, and productive person, exploring can add considerable value to your life.

Live with less

Simplification can dramatically change many aspects of your life. You don't have to be minimalist. You just have to be more aware of your purchasing options and think about your purchasing habits. At the same time, you will become less dependent on the acquisition of material goods.

Create routines

Morning and afternoon routines are very similar to the concept of overlapping habits. By establishing routines, you prepare your mind and body for the next day or night of rest. This is a great way to get into the right state of mind quickly.

Enjoy the sunrise or sunset

When was the last time you enjoy the beauty of sunrise or sunset? It is a truly fantastic experience, but we often ignore it. Don't take this fantastic experience for granted.

Live in the present

Let's be honest; the past cannot be changed. At the same time, it is not possible to predict the future. All we have is this moment, right now! This is the opportunity we have to do everything possible to build a better future. But most of the time, we find ourselves deeply obsessed with the past or concerned with the future. It is an unfortunate situation because it cancels the power of the present moment.

Developing new habits can be a daunting task. There will be many excuses, and at the same time, many old behavior patterns will resurface. Don't give up, be patient, and follow your new behavior. Once you cross the threshold, you will see these new habits will emerge. You will find yourself almost automatically absorbed by the latest patterns you acquired, and this is where most of the battle ends.

Conclusion

There are many reasons why someone should use hypnosis to lose weight. First, hypnosis is often successful when all other avenues of weight, health, and fitness have failed, and that's for a good reason!

The problem is not the method or even the plan you are using to achieve it. The problem is in your mind. If you want to lose real body fat, reduce weight, make your ideal shape, and maintain your new look, it is essential to change your attitude towards food and exercise, and your behavior towards both.

The best hypnosis programs for weight loss may require you to understand and replicate those mental processes used by people who have lost weight already. It might be tough leaving your comfort zone, but hypnosis will help you to reprogram your mind and install new thoughts that will become automatic habits once you identify the right behavior perfect for achieving your goal.

Eating less and adequately, or exercise following a schedule won't be a dream anymore: hypnosis enhances and strengthens your will.

So, if you are worried about being overweight now, there is nothing wrong with undergoing hypnosis. After all, you have nothing to lose but weight.